D1565184

3 STEPS TO THE MILLION-DOLLAR PRACTICE

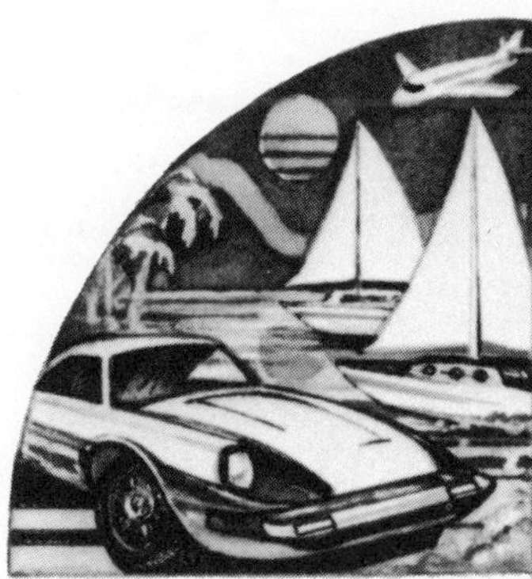
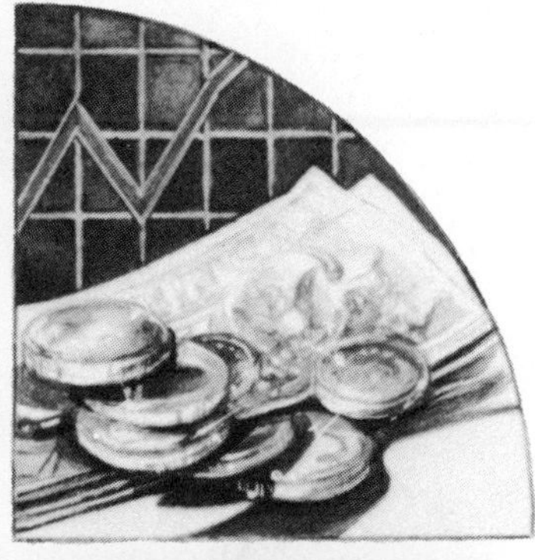
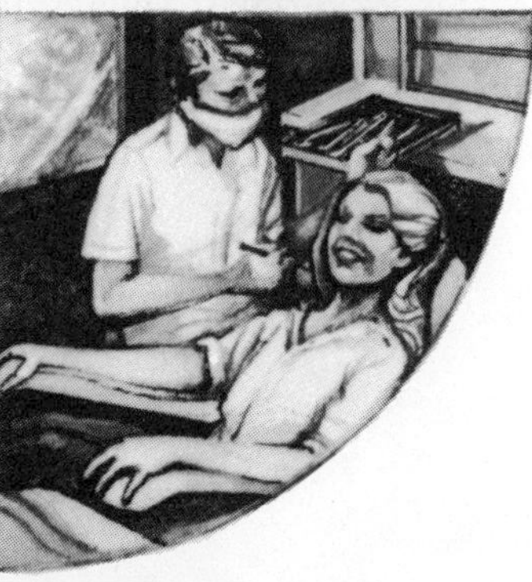

3 Steps to the Million-Dollar Practice

Duane A. Schmidt, DDS

PennWell Books

Dental Economics

PennWell Publishing Company
Tulsa, Oklahoma

To Cyndee and Cathy, the most beautiful programs of my Life.

Also by Duane A. Schmidt
THE LATE J.C.

by PennWell Publishing Co.,
1421 S. Sheridan Road/P. O. Box 1260
Tulsa, OK 74101

Library of Congress cataloging in publication data

Schmidt, Duane A.
3 steps to the million-dollar practice.

Includes index.
1. Dentistry—Practice. 2. Dentistry—Practice—Finance. I. Title.
II. Title: Three steps to the million-dollar practice.

RK58.S37 1985 617.6'0068 84-14765
ISBN 0-87814-266-5

Printed in the United States of America

CONTENTS

THANK YOU

Many hands and heads were involved in putting together this book. I want to thank them because they are special people.

Thank you, Dr. Joe Dunlap, for your powerful drive, your knack of turning clumsy wording into well-oiled verbiage, and your faith in seeing this book in print. Mostly, thanks for inspiring me to see the hope at the end of the tunnel.

Thank you, Kathryne Pile, editorial director of PennWell Books. Without your keen insight, beautiful suggestions, and dedication to bringing quality materials to the profession, there would be no need to thank anyone else—at least not for a finished book.

Thank you, Dr. George Layman, for a full measure of your thoughtful review and inspiring suggestions.

Thank you, Melvin J. Goldberg, for copyediting portions of this manuscript. I have always liked the way you tighten mediocrities into something more.

Thank you, Dr. Irving Bennet, without whose inspiration (read that "hammerlock") I would not have codified these thoughts. Many speaking engagements later these words bubbled up.

Thank you, Marla Wardell, for typing your little fingers raw as we went through draft after draft.

Thank you, Arthur and Eunice Schmidt (God bless his soul and rest hers), for having the courage to bring me into this century and teach me values that are comfortable to live with.

Thank you, Steve Williams, for programming me (with my own program yet!) to get off my duff and share this with others. I wanted to keep it to myself. I gave Steve every hackneyed excuse in the world for not writing it out. He would have none of it. He just used his hackney saw and lopped them off.

Thank you, *Dental Economics, Dental Management,* and *Dental Practice,* for generously allowing use of previously published articles of mine.

Thanks to my generous and gracious friends who allowed an intrusion on their demanding schedules to preview this manuscript. Thank you, Neil Brahe, Paul Jacobi, Omer Reed, Bob Levoy, Jim Rhode, Mel Goldberg, Irv Bennet, Jack Runninger, Barry Block, Peter Fernandez, Bob Williams, and Susan Bunnell. Your encouragement has been heartening.

Thank you, Editor Carolin Middleton of PennWell Books, who has mastered the art and science of syntax polishing and author embarrassment prevention. If this book sings, she was at least the lead soloist.

Thank you, Dr. Doug Nelson, who showed me that PASSION! was possible. And thanks to my former wet-fingered teachers who have since gone to that great beyond: Herbie Hoover, Ken Wessels, Bill Goodale, Gerry Scheckel, Bill Mellerup, and Frank Molsberry. Their wisdom lives and serves me to this day.

Finally, thanks to all those dentists whom I have looked up to and learned from during these thirty years of wet fingers.

Scaling the Mountain

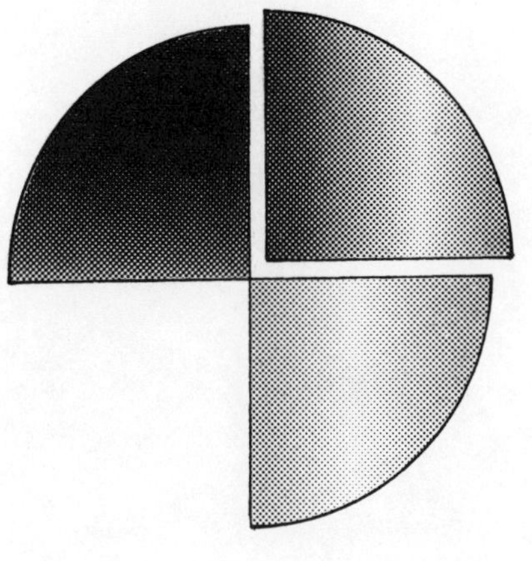

SECTION I:

1 INTRODUCTION

To get to the top of an oak tree, plant an acorn and sit on it . . . or climb an oak tree!

—*Anon.*

In Biblical times a man and his boy were leading their donkey down a path. The path was strewn with sharp rocks that cut their sandals and caused their feet to bleed.

Some people at the side of the road saw them and shouted: "Hey, old man. Why don't you ride your donkey?"

The man stopped. "Of course, of course," he muttered and mounted the animal. They walked along until they happened onto another group of people who shouted: "Hey, old man! Your boy's feet are bleeding. How come you are riding and he is walking?"

The man stopped. "Of course, of course," he mumbled. He dismounted and lifted his boy on the donkey. They walked on. Soon they passed still another group of people who shouted: "Hey, old man! You have a big, healthy donkey. Why aren't you *both* riding?"

"Good heavens! They are right," the man said, and so he mounted the donkey with his boy. The donkey trudged on.

Soon they came to a river. Recent rains had caused the river to rise and the current to be swift and treacherous. A narrow bridge was strung across the river. The donkey bearing the old man and his boy started across the bridge above the raging waters.

When they reached the middle of the river, the bridge collapsed. The man, boy, and donkey were plummeted into the vicious current.

Because they were rested from the ride, the old man and his boy were able to struggle to shore. But the donkey, being tired from his hard journey, was swept to his death.

The moral of the story is this: *He who tries to follow everyone's advice may one day lose his ass!*

Today we use other than the Biblical term for a donkey, but the moral holds true. If we followed all the advice that floods our dental offices, we might drown like the donkey.

Once upon a time, I burned out in dentistry. There was little satisfaction, not as much fulfillment as I thought there should be, not the growth or challenge I felt equal to, and small hope for the future.

Financially, the practice was a success. Emotionally, it was not. So I sold out and stood back for a couple of years and looked dentistry over. During that time I developed a program that needed testing.

In 1975 I opened a general practice with one employee and no patients in a toughly competitive dental market. Today, we have thirty employees, two associates, and over 6,000 square feet of office space. The program worked.

It can for you, too.

2
A DIFFERENT KIND OF ANIMAL

A mind stretched by a new idea never returns to its original dimension.

—Anon.

Last winter after an exhilarating day on the ski slopes, we joined the aprés crowd at Vail. The toddies were gentle, the atmosphere toasty and laidback. Steve and I toasted our good fortune.

"How come you *always* answer 'Super!' whenever anyone asks what kind of a day you're having, Schmidty?" Steve asked.

"Well that's how I program a super day," I said.

"But don't you ever have a bad day?" he asked.

"Nope. Tried one once and didn't like it."

Steve laughed. "Seriously, don't you really have days when you just want to throw in the towel?"

"Steve, who in the world doesn't? But I try to program a good day from the first crack I get at it. They mostly turn out that way," I answered.

"What's with programming?" Steve asked.

We worked on that until "last call" drove us into the icy streets. We talked about programming and how it is as simple as one, two, three. Steve vowed to program me to write it out. He succeeded.

* * *

In an age when a great deal of paper is covered with descriptions of how ape-like man is, little discussion goes on about how he differs from baboons and their cousins. Charles Darwin admitted that the "chasm between the intellect of the most intelligent ape and the least intelligent human may be fatal to this theory." Charles Darwin has a lot of company in contemplating that chasm.

It staggers the imagination to believe that man evolved from the apes. (If he did, it sometimes seems the ape got the best of the bargain.)

One of the chief arguments of Dr. Darwin's theory was his idea that various cultures of man have differing degrees of intellect. Primitive, tribal cultures were at the low end of the scale, and Western civilizations—to which Dr. Darwin belonged, naturally—were at the high end. He learned this "fact" from missionaries he'd met on his world voyage.

They were wrong, Charlie! Most anthropologists today agree that Australian aborigines and African pygmies, for example, have the same intellectual potential as civilized man. Having different roots doesn't mean being intellectually inferior. That's true whether you eat a missionary for lunch or take him to "21." The son of a jungle chieftain could graduate from Harvard magna cum laude, alongside the tycoon's daughter, given the proper rich daddy.

There doesn't seem to be much evidence to indicate that man's intellect has improved over the ages. The earliest known alphabet is far more complex than the one that blankets these pages. Astronomers knew the earth was round before the days of Christ. They had even measured it to within a few feet of the size modern scientists claim the earth to be. A computer has been recovered from the wreck of a ship off the shore of Greece. The shipwreck occurred decades before Christ lived. And Moses' great grandparents, as well as his children, had about the same kinds of problems we do.

The consensus today seems to be: Man's intellect arrived on the scene fullblown; it hasn't changed much through time. And while various cultures may peer through different-colored glasses, they use a remarkably similar intellect when deciding whether to kill their neighbor with a spear or a .45.

What is this universal piece of original equipment man carries about in his head that's called intellect? I don't have enough to know. I'm not sure anyone does. Scientists still have their hands full trying to put the difference between being asleep and being awake into words that anyone, including themselves, can understand.

There is, however, a corollary with something modern man does understand—the computer. Now the word "understand" is a funny word. I don't really understand a computer in the sense that I know what happens within its bowels. I don't.

But I can *appreciate* what it does, and that is all that really matters. I also don't "understand" a sunrise, a musical comedy, or love. But I like what they do for me, and that's enough for me to know about them.

A computer can do two things:

1. Calculate, that is, add and subtract, and
2. Move information.

Before a computer performs those tasks, it must be given a list of directions called a program. Once programmed, it will mechanically perform its designated tasks in tiny fractions of seconds. It does them over and again, without complaint, never asking for a raise or time off to go to traffic court with Junior. Computers never become pregnant nor demand a "Take Your Computer to Lunch Week." That's all we need to know about computers.

Intellect compares with computer functions in that our response to a situation is determined by *our programs*. We receive input or perception of situations through our five senses, much like data are fed into a computer by a keypunch operator.

Once we perceive, we respond according to the directions contained in our programs. That's how our intellect is computer-like. We differ from computers in that: (1) We have control of our programs; (2) we establish priorities in choosing which of several actions to take; and (3) we can push our own starter button.

The difference is marvelous for it means we can program ourselves for whatever we choose. We control our own programs. But we can allow others to influence the nature of our programs. We can accept or deny others' programs, just as we can attempt to reprogram those with whom we have influence. Thus is created the exquisite opportunity for man to be the most unique animal on this third planet from the sun.

We are unique because we can program our computer-like intellects—call it brain, mind, or intellect—to respond to our wishes.

To create a successful program, three steps are mandatory:

1. We must know the rules required by whatever program we choose;
2. We must be willing to take a risk; and most importantly,
3. We must pursue our goal with PASSION!

A pleasant discovery is that we already know how to program ourselves. We do it all the time. We have done it for years, knowingly and unknowingly. But we don't need to know *how* to do it as much as we need to know *why* we do it. And we also need to know how to channel our own programming into successful veins.

To program a computer would take you long hours of study. Our task may not be that difficult. When you have finished this book, you should possess all you need to program yourself for personal victories in and out of your dental office.

One of the reasons we are already familiar with the programming process is that it began the instant the sperm zapped the ovum that produced us.

Back when we were about the size of a dot on the letter "i," we were already programmed in many ways. The color of our eyes, skin, and hair was already determined. So was the length of our arms and legs and torso. Our predisposition to disease, the number of our bicuspids, and our absorption rate of Vitamin C were also included in that little dot. Incredible! One incredible, little dot!

We are stuck with the programs in the dot just as we are stuck with the fact the dot may have resided in an endometrium in Buckingham palace or a grass shack in Boro Boro. That doesn't mean, however, that we have to stay in the palace or grass shack—just in the endometrium and only there for a while.

It also doesn't mean we have to live life as a redhead or bald head if we don't want to. We are what we become. Programming is all about learning to do more with what we are given in the first place. And we can because each of us was dealt a multibillion-dollar piece of equipment—a brain.

As the little dot grows, countless programs begin to function. Soon it is launched into society. Its billion programs continue to operate. There's scarcely enough paper in the world to describe all the physiological reactions necessary for a baby to smile, suck his thumb, or pass gas. They are so complex and so handsomely preprogrammed from the very outset. It's all so terribly convenient.

Baby quickly learns there are many more universal programs in store for him. The laws of gravity, algebra, and Yin and Yang fall on the just and the unjust alike. A skinned nose means the same in every language. But these laws are all conveniently preprogrammed from day one. In time, baby learns to sort his way through them. And he also learns that a skinned nose usually heals.

As he grows, he learns that even more programs have been laid out for him by his culture and society. He learns it isn't cool to pick his nose in public. He learns to control the sphincters of his orifices, both mouth and otherwise.

He learns to communicate. And he learns that the law of gravity has a mirror image that is equally compelling—the gravity of the law.

All of these programs are standard equipment. He can do little to change them. It is into this maze of programs that Little Dots grow and prosper—or suffer. But we haven't mentioned his companions on this journey—his parents, peers, and other people contacts.

Depending on which shift they work, parents spend a great deal of time parenting. What they attempt to do is program Little Dot to become like them, or hopefully, better. Their likes and dislikes often become his. Their values, traditions, and opinion of

Teddy Kennedy become his, too. So do their hopes, fears, and ability to love.

His peers attempt to do the same thing. They want him to develop a proper fear of bullies, a proper reverence for P.S. 122, and a proper ability to slouch about in slovenly garb.

His people contacts lay a few more programs on him in an attempt to program him to respect Chaucer, logarithms, and escargot.

Sooner or later—sometimes never—Little Dot learns that some of the programs that were foisted on him are faulty. He learns that which every computer scientist has embroidered on his shorts: GIGO—garbage in, garbage out. If incorrect information is fed into a computer, the computer can neither correct it or shove it around the chips in any reasonable manner at all.

Ben Franklin fed the world a line about a penny saved being a penny earned. Little Dot believed that at first. He believed it until he watched inflation wipe out Grandpa's pennies. And maybe, just maybe, he realized one day that every billionaire who ever died was struggling to make another buck the moment he gave up the struggle.

Or perhaps he learns that the only thing people learn from failure is how to fail. Maybe he learns that a nose to the grindstone is apt to produce a ground-off nose and no success at all. Or maybe he will spend his entire life arguing about what success means or if it means anything at all.

Bewildered by all this, Little Dot may wander about unprogrammed, trying to withdraw from everyone's attempts to program him to support either Planned Parenthood or Unplanned Parenthood.

And so all of us Little Dots arrive at today, simply a collection of our yesterdays. But if that is true—and it seems reasonably apparent that it is—then our tomorrows can be whatever we want them to be.

Earl Nightingale says we are what we want to be. Perhaps more accurately, we are not what we want to be today, but what we wanted to be yesterday. To me, this implies greater hope. Because it presents the opportunity for us to become whatever we want to program ourselves to become tomorrow.

Our todays become the tomorrows we programmed yesterday. Our tomorrows will become whatever we program today. Got that? Okay, let's see how it works.

3
EXODUS FROM TODAY

God didn't take the time to make nobody.

—Zig Ziglar

God was so tickled when He made you that He made only one of you. And that goes double for twins. If He didn't want you to be anything more than your genetic programs, He could easily have left out intellect and simply made more monkeys.

You are not an accident of nature, Darwinian myopia to the contrary. We are carefully planned people who have the delightful luxury of making our marvelous programming ability produce extraordinary results.

For results to happen, our plan must be valid. We cannot change the color of our skin, but we can learn a new language. We cannot change our parents, but we can change the way we are parents. We cannot change our height, but we can surely change our stature among men.

About everything else can be changed. While we may not like certain things about our life, we have to like ourselves, for starters. We have to appreciate the beauty of life, the hope of tomorrow, and the joy of sharing a jot of this journey with others whom God was happy He created.

For programmed changes to occur, three things must happen: (1) You must *know* the rules; (2) you must be willing to risk success; and (3) you must play the game with PASSION! Let's see how we can use these concepts.

1. *Know the rules.* We must develop an intellectual awareness. We gotta' know the rules. You cannot program yourself to become a surgeon unless you know the foreign language that goes on about the body, unless you receive all the proper parchments, and like Doonesbury says, unless you know your tax shelters.

"Do you play the piano?" she asked.

"I don't know, I never tried," he answered.

He couldn't, of course; he didn't know the rules. He could program a friend to play for his enjoyment. Or he could program himself to earn enough to hire a pianist or go to a concert or purchase a tape cassette. Or he could spend the effort to learn the rules.

Consider the recent dental graduate who hungers for success. He may think he knows the rules, but we all recall how little we really knew about the management of a practice, about communication, and about money matters back when we ached our way through those lonely days.

Consider the experienced generalist who longs for specialty status. How empty will that longing be until he learns to bend the wire, thread the canal, slice the gum tissue, or whatever specialty he seeks? He may know many rules, but he doesn't know those special set of credentials that specialists hold themselves to and that other generalists demand of the specialties.

Two cautions need repeating about knowing the rules. The first is to recognize that there is no avoiding this step in *any* program. If it is for financial success in dentistry, then you must know the rules for that. If it is for investment success in commodity trading, then you must know the rules for that. Although many try, there is no way to succeed without knowing the rules.

Many dentists believe that since they know the rules for success in dentistry they are, therefore, shrewd enough to succeed at any other game—even when they don't know how to play the other game. How vain. Pride goeth before a fall?

But learning the rules is the phase that many would like to avoid. It's work, enormously profitable, but still mind-sapping work. You will avoid paying income taxes easier than you can avoid step one. Without mastering step one there are no steps two and three.

The second caution is that knowing the rules does not, of itself, guarantee success *unless* you go to steps two and three. All geniuses are not wealthy.

Mensa is an American organization for people in the top 2% IQ. We call them geniuses. Yet, in this elite organization there are expansive rules to help the many geniuses in America who cannot afford the $30 annual dues! How does it feel to be wealthier than many geniuses? I know, nice.

A person may be the finest dentist, attorney, or concert pianist in the world, but unless he goes to steps two and three, it means nothing. He may be spending his days either slicing beef tenderloins at Sardi's or bruising beef tenderloins with the Dallas Cowboys. Knowing the rules simply isn't enough. There must be a:

2. *Willingness to risk.* The Cowboys don't feel supremely confident going into every game, and neither does the TMJ expert when he faces an unruly bite nor the pianist as he faces the music.

Willingness to apply the rules means becoming an active participant. You must be willing to stick your neck out and take a chance. That means being willing to risk falling on your face. A game never played is never lost. Neither is it ever won. But there is cuddly comfort in fantasizing how great the results would be "*if* I did this or that."

Mr. Doug Amway—no relation to *the* Mr. Amway—didn't win his pink Cadillac selling Mary Kay products by daydreaming. He could know MK's product line like he knows which spots on Mrs. Amway's back feel best when he gives her her nightly rub. But knowing isn't enough. And that's the rub.

Practice-management experts report that most new dentists, after they have made a beautiful presentation and demonstrated how well they know their product, forget to ask the customer to buy. Do they "forget"? Or do they not ask because by not asking for a "yes" they never risk hearing a "no"? I suspect the fear of failure deters more sales than any other single factor.

Not only does it block sales, but fear of failure stops plays from being written, songs from being composed, dates from being asked for, and Mary Kay Krumplestein from realizing her full potential as an Amway distributor because she's afraid of the possibility of losing a sale.

A loser is not a person who tries and fails. A loser is a person who never tries at all.

Babe Ruth, the Sultan of Swat, struck out 1,732 times. Had he never gone to bat, he would not have sliced so much air with his Louisville Slugger. He also would not have gone down in history as the Homerun King. Hank Aaron, who broke Babe's record, struckout more times than 99% of the ballplayers in the major leagues!

Frankly, it would be quite comfortable talking about this book, rather than having a go at it. The world is full of people who call themselves authors, who are "working on a book," and who will never publish. They cannot risk bombing out with a bummer.

Failing to risk failure, they embrace an even greater failure—doing nothing at all. What's the old saying about love? *Better to have loved and lost than to have never loved at all.* Better to have tried and failed than to have never tried at all. But that takes persistence and determination.

Author Unknown wrote it:

Press On

> Nothing in the world takes the place of persistence and determination.
> Talent will not. Unsuccessful men with talent are legion.
> Genius will not. Unrewarded genius is proverb.
> Education will not. The world is full of educated derelicts.
> Persistence and determination alone are omnipotent.

Thomas Edison failed 14,000 times before he invented the incandescent light bulb. Someone asked if that bothered him. "*No,*" he replied, "I didn't fail 14,000 times. I successfully found 14,000 ways that didn't work," Now that's a winner's attitude.

We might say, "Sure. But look how successful he became when he got it right." That is true. But he didn't know he would succeed when he tried his 14,000th unsuccessful test. He kept right on doggedly determined, convinced that genius was, in his words, "1% inspiration and 99% perspiration."

Operatic star Enrico Caruso's teacher told him to give up music, since he failed to hit so many high notes. Albert Einstein and Werner Von Braun both flunked courses in math. Vince Lombardi was still a line coach at Fordham at age 43. Walt Disney went broke seven times and had a nervous breakdown before he drew Mickey Mouse.

Examples of outstanding successes are not difficult to cite. In each case they first learned the rules of the game they wanted to play. Then they had the courage to play the game. But they also had one more ingredient that made them a head taller than anyone else in the ballpark. They had:

3. *PASSION!* A passion to play with all the equipment they possessed. Passion sets winners apart from also-rans. Passion is not "I wish . . ." or even "I want to . . ."; it is "I will!" Winners know that the difference between the leader and the rest of the pack is only a tiny fraction.

Wilhelm Reiss, a German inventor, perfected a device for transmitting sound over a wire years before anyone else had the idea. Had he moved two electrodes 1/1000 of an inch closer, he would have invented the telephone.

Several years later, an obscure college professor spent all his spare time and dollars trying to find a way to help his hard-of-hearing wife with her problem. He failed, but we remember Alexander Graham Bell for his momentous discovery of the telephone.

PASSION! The most powerful word in the English language. It's the possession of all people with the power to achieve; the steam that drives the engine of the mind to accomplish whatever task it addresses; the generator that turns mere life into a thrilling, living experience. Passion!

The world is filled with people who understand that intellectual awareness must precede any beneficial change in lifestyle. But most people stop there, bemoaning the fact that the world does not give them the recognition they feel is there due for their education, their talent, or even their genius. Knowing the rules is simply not enough. No one ever improved his lot by reading a self-help book nor even by memorizing it. Improvement comes from applying that which has been read.

There are an oh-so-few who not only know the rules and are willing to risk failure, but who also embrace life with passion. Their successes are dizzying to the hordes.

They know how to experience joy in their love affair with life. And that's what PASSION! is all about.

4
THE TOUGHEST SALE IN THE WORLD

All you need to succeed is a fancy car, a good address, and a suntan.

—Aristotle Onassis

Billy Graham, Carl Sagan, and Jack LaLane have a lot in common. Their names are readily recognized in their various fields of endeavor. They bear the accoutrements of success. However, their areas of expertise differ markedly, each being associated with a different aspect of man: his spirit, mind, and body.

It might seem that one of these areas—spirit, mind, or body—must receive paramount attention if we're to achieve fulfillment as a human being. But if we were to adopt that narrow view of those disciplines, we would be afflicted with the most common eye disease in the world—tunnel vision.

We each own a spirit, mind, and body. But they must work in concert. A conductor who addresses only the flute section isn't going to orchestrate much music out of the brass and the strings. And his drummers may miss the beat entirely.

We recognize that sanctification of the spirit is the longest term goal of all, and we understand that the marvels of the mind can make it all happen; however, unless we have a body that works, not much else matters. Dying is a certain way to end all programs. And dying early is a tacky thing to do; it's such a waste of the glories that could have been.

Living a long time is a nice thing to do. A long life is even better if it is productive, abundant, and fulfilled. Having the physical plant to make that happen is surely a pleasant prospect. But there is another benefit to being in a good physical shape. It's called making a good first impression.

The first squawk we let out on planet earth is an attempt to sell someone on the idea of providing us with food, love, and tender care. Even our last gasp, when we are trying to interest someone in remembering us, is an attempt to *sell. Every waking hour of every day of our lives we attempt to sell something to someone.*

Almost all the sales we make stem from the first impressions we deliver. Sales experts agree that 80% of the people who turn away from a sale do so because of the seller's (doctor's) appearance. Eighty percent!

With millions of people who have something to sell vying for the attention of millions of others, there isn't time for lengthy examinations. We make quick decisions as to whether or not we'll enter relationships, try products, or simply keep bumping along watching for the next opportunities.

It may not be fair, but that's the way it is. Maybe people should not judge a book by its cover, but they do. Do you believe, even for a moment, that some high-priced art talent was not hired to produce the cover on this book? You know better than that and so does the publisher.

Ari Onassis was saying the same thing in Golden Greek style in his quote at the beginning of this section.

Looks do make the man, and the woman. Robert Redford, Paul Newman, Ann-Margret, and Jane Fonda recognize this. They know that an attractive person, properly packaged, is a highly marketable asset. If you don't believe this is true for the rest of us, then you seriously underestimate human behavior.

Is good human packaging to create a good first impression a ploy, a sham, deceitful, or misleading? Not at all. For you will make a first impression whether or not you shave, shower, and shampoo. It will just be a different kind of first impression.

The term "first impression" is misleading. There are no second impressions. We are lucky to get one shot. If we fluff that, we can forget having a second opportunity. Advertisers call this the "10 to 1 Rule."

Introduce a product, an idea, or a person to a marketplace and—for the sake of illustration—say it costs you $1. Try to reintroduce that product, idea, or person for a second impression, and it will cost $10. That's an unhealthy difference in cost. But it emphasizes the value—and power—of a good first impression.

Dr. Robert Carlton at the University of Iowa has found in a study of first impressions that people remember an impression long after they have forgotten the events of that impression. He found that the tone of a person's voice, his stature, physical appearance, and eye contact had 65% more bearing on a first impression than what a person said or did!

In a copyrighted story in *Cue New York* (January 19, 1979) Jacqueline Thompson writes:

> Many psychologists and sociologists have embarked on studies to determine the role physical attractiveness plays in a person's life. Based on a variety of experiments and tests, these researchers have already come to the preliminary conclusion that the *comely constitute a privileged caste in this country and enjoy advantages based solely on the external attributes willed to them in the genetic sweepstakes. . . .* (italics mine)
>
> The University of Minnesota's Dr. Ellen Bersheid, for instance, has found evidence of a "Strong physical attractiveness stereotype." She claims attractive people are assumed to be "kinder, more genuine, sincere, warm, sexually responsive, poised, modest, sociable, sensitive, interesting, strong, more exciting, more nurturant, and of better character than the less handsomely endowed."

Whew! Packaging ourselves for life's adventures begins with taking stock of the shape we are in. Have you got enough you to do the job and not too much to hold you back? Is the you that you've got in good working order, able to physically handle the demands you want your you to do?

Most of us need to get leaner. That must be true because diet books routinely weigh down bestseller lists. Most of them are disguised starvation programs, designed to allow their readers to have their cake and eat it, too—weight-lossly. *All you lose on a 30-day crash diet is one month.*

Or have you fallen victim to fables about fat? Fat people are jolly. Fat people have more fun. There's more of you to love. Fat is beautiful. Have you fallen for the Twinkie mentality that's loose in the land today? Joe pats his paunch and says, "It's mine, and it's all paid for!"

You're half right, Joe. It's yours, to be sure, but it isn't all paid for. You pay for it in countless ways every day.

Fat shortens your stamina and ability to perform, just as surely as it shortens your life. It clots your arteries, overburdens your heart, and holds you back from everything—including the plate you so frequently reach for.

No, Joe. Sorry. You haven't begun to pay for a paunch that saddles your life like it saddles your waist.

An excellent reprogramming method for your emergence is exercise. To be productive, exercise should elevate the heartbeat, cause us to sweat for fifteen minutes, increase breathing, and employ as many muscles as possible. Golf and bowling, fun though they may be, do not qualify.

Tennis and racquetball fulfill the requirements, as do jogging and swimming laps—if you are really into boredom, that is. Vigorous sport helps awaken sleepy fat so that it is burned off.

A friend told me recently the three characteristics to look for in choosing a doctor. He should have grey hair to look distinguished, wear glasses to look intelligent, and have hemorrhoids—so he has the proper look of concern about the patient's problems!

I'll settle for a lean doctor. Overweight doctors disturb me, just as do overweight clergy, motivationists, and dieticians.

With the physical reprogrammed, we can turn to the mind. A body tuned up needs a mind turned on. Let's visit Passion U.

5 PASSION! U.

A rut is just a casket with the ends knocked out.

—Lowell Lundstrom

A few years ago a Midwesterner went West where a hot little business caught his eye. He bought in, then bought out his partners, and soon began franchising his operation thoughout the country.

Early on he realized that his franchisees needed to know more than how to mix the meat and light the oven. He realized they had to sell. To reprogram them for greater success, he established Hamburger University in a suburb of Chicago.

The wisdom of his effort has not been lost on his business, for through his golden arches have marched 45 billion Big and little Macs.

Would it be possible to reprogram ourselves at PASSION U. to have a zest for living equal to the zeal MacDonald franchisees have for selling sesame-seed buns? If we did, the curriculum might look something like this.

Interest & Enthusiasm 101

Have you ever heard someone enjoying a hearty laugh, the kind we call a belly laugh? Did you want to join in it? If the laugh went on long enough, you probably did.

Certain people who have an infectious laugh make you want to laugh whenever you hear theirs. A few people with that capacity even earn their living as professional laughers, being spotted throughout an audience to inspire people to let go and laugh.

Enthusiasm is about like that because enthusiasm breeds more enthusiasm. Don't you feel a warmth when you visit with people who have bright and sunny dispositions? Don't you like sharing their happiness, being in the sunlight they cast? We all do.

Your enthusiasm reprograms people around you. They become more responsive, less negative, brighter, happier, and more friendly when they catch your spirit of enthusiasm. It's the old saw about giving away a smile and getting back more than you gave because you still have your own at the end of the day. That's a bargain on which you can't lose.

Or are you stuck in a rut, wishing your life away? "Gee I wish it were Friday." "Gee, I wish it were summer." "Gee, I wish it weren't raining."

Lowell Lundstrom points out that when we are 30 we only have 2,000 weeks left before we are boxed! And when we are 50, we only have 1,000 weeks left! That's not much time, brothers and sisters. Are you wishing those few weeks away?

Enthusiasm is the daughter of PASSION! and the bride of interest. Are they your relatives? Not bad folks to have around. And they can be programmed without all that much effort. We each have the power to attain those benefits.

Or are you stuck in a TV rut? The last game of the World Series ended, and she snapped off the set with a sigh. She set out a bottle of wine, slipped into a negligee, and cuddled up to him on the sofa.

"Gee, you look nice, Honey. But I didn't know you had a grey negligee," he said.

"I don't," she answered. "It's dust!"

But interest and enthusiasm aren't enough. We also need Positive Thinking 202.

Positive Thinking 202

How many times have you heard: "Well, it's human nature to ______." Fill in the missing blank. This is one of the classic cop-outs. If "human nature" means it is what most people do, then it is human nature to be overweight, malnourished, mentally impoverished, and unsuccessful. The last thing we who want to change ourselves need is a negative program. And self-inflicted negative programs are suicidal to success, the worst cut of all.

Perhaps no other single event in our lives demonstrates the power of programming like these negative programs. Jeff has a cousin of whom most everyone in the family says: "Oh, Janey always loses things." Well, sure enough, Janey responds by losing things. Janey is caught in the web of a negative program just as surely as is another of his relatives who is programmed to be 150 pounds overweight—"Oh, Billy has this enormous appetite."

A lady wanted to borrow a cup of sugar, so she started next door with an empty cup in hand. Along the way she began thinking: "My neighbor will really think it's dumb of me to have to borrow a cup of sugar, She's got so much, and we've got so little. She's got a Mercedes in her driveway, and all we've got is a Pinto. She has a real pool in her backyard, and we're lucky to have a plastic wader. She belongs to a country club, and we can't even afford a book club. Boy, is she going to laugh at me!"

When she arrived at her neighbor's door, she had worked up a pretty good tizzy. Her neighbor answered the doorbell: "Oh, hi. May I help you?" she asked.

The lady threw down her cup and said; "Keep your darned old sugar!"

Reprogramming your computer starts with yourself. It's "I can do," "I am important in God's plan for this world or else why would He have made me?" "I have the power to do anything I set my program to do, because I own the world's most beautiful computer—my mind."

The positive-thinking program extends to those about you. "Super" sets the pace. People know you are turned on, going places, doing things, and not going to wishy-wash your way through life. Your power becomes evident and produces real results.

Court friends who reinforce your positive program. Surround your life with winners because you want to win at whatever you set out to do. Let the negatives slide out of your life. Sure, it is difficult to "fire" a friend, but sometimes it must be done if they negatively affect your life.

Robert J. Ringer in his bestseller *Looking Out for Number One* said:

> There are certain things you cannot change, don't let them occupy your valuable time or thought. Your parentage, for example, the color of your skin, the Mid-East crisis, interest rates, and so on. Since you cannot do one blooming thing about them, why waste any effort on them?

Good point. We can't do a thing about the cold war, California earthquakes and mudslides, oil company profits, the arms race, or headline hunting scientists with scare stories about cancer being caused by lipstick, cranberries, saccharine, or margarine. So let's not waste an erg of our energy pining for what might have been and for what we cannot influence.

I recently refused a reviewer to reprogram my day. I had delivered a talk in Los Angeles. Afterward, the audience filled out reviews, so the sponsors might determine if I should be invited back.

The person wrote my nickname on the page—a one word statement about my talk. Strange! Even more strange, you would think an educated person would know how to spell "Schmitty." He didn't. Sonofogun, he left out the "M"!

Let's refuse to be like the lady going for the cup of sugar, and say: "Life is full of Hell. So keep your old life!" Nosiree. Life is gorgeous and our cup is half full, not half empty.

With these two courses in hand, we turn to Philosophy 303.

Philosophy 303

I don't know what tomorrow holds, but I know *Who* holds tomorrow. You do, too. We must have a philosophy to function, or there is no reason to function. *The purpose for being is to become a being with a purpose.* We must operate from a credo, which in turn must match the plan of the universe if it is to work at all.

A man who shoots his mother-in-law at 500 yards may be considered a good shot, if not much of a man. Come to think of it, that sentence was probably a cheap shot at mothers-in-law. Sorry about that.

I won't lay my philosophy of life on you if you will return the favor. My philosophy probably only works for me, anyway, just as yours does for you. Suffice it to say that we each need a philosophy to make life worthwhile.

Some years ago the Navy thrust me into a clinic with a group of dentists from various parts of the country. One of them became a friend, and I asked him why he never did an MOD.

"No percentage," he replied.

"I don't understand. What do you mean by that?"

"Well, if you do an MO and later a DO you get to charge more than for an MOD."

I hope dentists with philosophies like that get slicked in business the same way they are slicking their patients. They deserve no better.

Goal Setting 404

The Rev. Robert Schuller says, "Failing to plan is planning to fail." And J.C. Penney once said, "Give me a stock clerk with goals, and I'll give you a man who will write history." Then he continued; "But give me a man without goals, and I'll give you a stock clerk."

Can you imagine Sir Edmund Hillary, the first man to conquer Mt. Everest, being asked how he got there and responding, "Well, we were just wandering around one day and found ourselves on top!"

Goal setting is the most visible of programming efforts we can make. A man without a goal is an actor without a script, a runner without a tape to cross, a quarterback without goalposts. What, for a quick example, is your goal in reading this book? Or are you wandering aimlessly through these pages, wondering what kind of a kook wrote it?

A pilot radioed a tower and asked for landing instructions. "Roger, where are you?" the air traffic controller answered.

"I don't know," said the pilot, "but I've got a whale of a tailwind, and we're making good time!"

Aren't we a lot like that a lot of time? We don't know where we are or where we're going but we've got a whale of a tailwind and we're making good time. But to where?

What about a goal of having financial security for life? Is that worthy of the efforts? Maybe. But what will you do with that pile of cash when you have it? Will you be happy? Will you be a better person? Will you be more worthy of respect? A better friend? Will you be assured a better afterlife? Will you be a better father, mother, sister, brother, son, daughter, neighbor, boss? How will it improve your lifestyle?

Mike, my accountant, told me the other day that I would leave exactly as much money as Howard Hughes. I became excited and asked Mike how much it would be.

"All of it," was his deadpan reply.

Having big bucks may change your lifestyle, but that isn't the point. Will it *improve* your lifestyle? An implication in that question is that you know what changes in your lifestyle would be an improvement. Do you?

If you had unlimited funds, what would you do then? Retire? To what? Buy expensive gifts for people? Afford expensive colleges for your children? Buy them all Porsches on their 21st birthdays? Buy grandma a floorlength mink? Tool around in a Ferrari? Just what is it you would do with great wealth that would create an improvement in you and your lifestyle? Change is not necessarily improvement.

Elvis Presley could buy things most people don't even know are for sale. But have you read of a more tormented life than his? As the seamy details of his life unfolded, the shallowness of monetary goals became apparent. The same can be said for Howard Hughes.

I'm not knocking financial success. But by itself, it's a pretty shallow goal. Surely there are great fruits of life to be enjoyed. We are promised, over and again, that they will be given to us "pressed down, shaken together, and overflowing."

Achieving monetary success is no more evil than being poor is virtuous. Sophie Tucker once said; "I've tried being rich, and I've tried being poor. Being rich is better."

A dentist friend of mine was obsessed with obtaining a million dollars. He worked 70–80 hours a week, missed most of the youth of his five children, never saw their school plays or sporting events. "Too busy! Sorry, kids. Daddy has to work tonight."

He got his million dollars, which his wife and her second husband are enjoying. Robert dropped dead a few months after he succeeded(?). Was his success worth the price he'd paid?

Our final course at PASSION! U. knits it all together with Persistence & Determination 505.

Persistence & Determination 505

The overriding program of every person who has ever succeeded at anything is rooted in persistence and determination, for these attributes alone are the final assurance of success. They are the heartbeat of PASSION!

No one who has succeeded at anything has done so without a passion for his effort. A casual wish is hardly a passion. "I wish I were this!" "I wish I had a thousand dollars!" "I wish I could take a year off and travel or study or go fishing!" It simply isn't enough.

Wishes are the thoughts of idle minds, playing with the toys of unfilled opportunities and unfulfilled dreams. PASSION! is a mind programmed so firmly that nothing can make it waver from its course; a mind that reprograms those around it to make its goals come true.

There was a man who wouldn't give up. His first business failed, but he didn't quit. He was defeated for the legislature, and his second business failed. Still he didn't quit. He suffered a nervous breakdown. Later he was defeated for speaker and for elector. He was twice defeated for Congress and once defeated for the Senate. But through it all, he hung in there; he didn't quit. He was defeated for vice president and defeated for the Senate again. Still he didn't quit.

Two years after his last election defeat, Abraham Lincoln became the 16th president of the United States. Abe Lincoln was a man with PASSION!

Super

How would you like to start a program working for you right this minute? It's fast and simple, and it works.

The next time someone asks, "Howya doin', Doc?" Answer, "Super!" That's all there is to the program! That's the entire program that gets pluses going where minuses used to dwell. It illustrates how simple it is to program a positive benefit.

Just this week I've met two new patients who even had that program whipped. The first said: "I'd have to have a relapse to be only fantastic!"

The second said: "The only way I could be better would be if I were twins!"

"Super!" is good enough. It tells your mind how you are going to be. Sure enough, your mind will hear it and respond. Lukewarm, mediocre living will liven up. Your juices will flow better, and those who hear your response will respond in kind.

Example: Did you ever ask someone how he was and he began a long litany of woe? Where did your mind shuffle off to? At least to Buffalo.

When they say "Oh, I guess I'll live." Check your immediate gut reaction. Bad, huh? Of course. They aren't even trying to program good, great, super.

What do you know about the person who says; "Guess I'll live?" You know, for certain, that he isn't really alive. Most of us treat those woebegoners accordingly. That's how people treat you when you come on flaccid.

It all depends on our priorities. If feeling super is important to you, then say it. All you gets is what you hears! If being super isn't a priority, then what priority would be important to you?

We choose our priorities from whatever we feel will bring us the greatest pleasure. Some people enjoy their ails and reject happiness because the only style they know is being miserable.

But you and I want better than that. We know that happiness is more fun. We know—or you will, as soon as you try the easy, "Super" program—that we can turn clouds into sunshine on our command.

Pleasure is the key. We have defined, and we constantly redefine, what brings us pleasure. Whatever it is, it will top our priority list at that moment.

For example, you walk into your office in the morning, "Good morning, Doctor," your employees greet you.

"Good morning!" you sing back to them, full of vibrance and meaning, looking them straight in the eye with a cheerful smile. With that you have begun to program your day. But then it happens.

Nancy enters your private office. "Doctor, the lab case for Mrs. Wilcox hasn't arrived and she's here now."

Two choices. Erupt with expletives over the lab's ineptitude or defuse this effort to reprogram your day.

"That's unfortunate. Call and find out why. Offer Mrs. Wilcox an explanation, an apology, and a cup of coffee, and let me know when the case will be here." Smile in a voice of calm measure.

Nancy finds the case is "on its way" and should be here in fifteen minutes.

"Thanks, Nancy. Mrs. Wilcox satisfied? Good. Now don't you think we should have a program where we check tomorrow's seatings today to see where the cases are?"

"Yes, doctor. I should have done that. I'll be sure it's done from now on."

"Thank you Nancy. Now let's have a super day."

Mrs. Wilcox is finally seated in the operatory.

"Mrs. Wilcox, I'm sorry your case arrived late, but you know that was a tricky one and I wanted to be sure it was 100% correct, not 98%. We just won't settle for anything less than the best for you."

The situation is handled, and you continue with your super day. Had you berated the lab for being late, chewed out Nancy for failing to perform properly, and laid the trip on Mrs. Wilcox, you would have negated an entire day's program in a few sentences.

It's sad, but true, that negatives can so easily gain control of our lives. In this simple, quick exchange, which is repeated thousands of times daily across the land, either a negative or positive benefit can occur. And either benefit is completely under the control of the doctor. Which do you want? How do *you* handle the late lab case syndrome?

A minor situation unworthy of comment? Hardly. Days are created by a series of such minor events, with people constantly trying to reprogram one another through the interplay of their words, attitudes, and actions.

If you want a super day, you have to go for it, cling to it, and not let anyone reprogram you—not a boorish driver in another car, not a supply house who backordered for the fortieth time, not a neglectful employee, not even a late lab case.

The story is told of a business magnate who with his friend stopped to buy a newspaper.

"Hi ya, Joe, how's it going?" The tycoon asked with a friendly smile.

The newsvendor swore and grunted an answer.

As they walked away, the businessman's friend asked, "How could you take that rotten answer and not answer in kind?"

The businessman replied: "I refuse to let a newsvendor control my day."

If misery is your thing, it isn't hard to program. If super is your goal, it's just as easy to program. But *we choose* which program we want, and that's what we get. We choose based upon what we believe will give us the greatest pleasure at that moment. Logic has nothing to do with it.

Is it logical to pay $20 an ounce for a cashmere sport coat or $5,000 for a carat diamond? Logic doesn't even enter into such decisions. They are made on the basis of what the buyer determines to be a pleasurable benefit.

Positive benefits can be programmed, as we noted in the Mrs. Wilcox episode, by the attitude of our actions. Perhaps a more vivid illustration of how we can program ourselves occurred in Dr. Raney's office.

The doctor was aware he had a problem in his office. His receptionist had a downright unfriendly voice. Patients had told him about it, he had heard it himself, and he knew that her "unsmiling" voice was costing him valuable first impressions. Where he should have been scoring points with callers, he was losing them. Discussing the problem with the young lady had only produced temporary improvements.

Then he read about a high school principal who had been faced with growing deportment problems among his students—beligerence in the classrooms, rowdiness in the halls, absenteeism, and sloppy dress. The principal decided to try something unique. It worked.

Shortly after he'd acted, these major problems with his students began to evaporate and things started getting back to normal.

What had he done? He had installed a huge mirror at the head of the stairs leading into the school. The students, seeing themselves, reprogrammed their behavior and normalcy returned.

Dr. Raney decided to try the same stunt. He installed a mirror in front of his receptionist's desk and said only one thing to her, "Smile, Connie." And Connie smiled. Her voice reflected the smile, and the practice basked in a happier glow.

If a simple expedient like a mirror can reprogram a student body and a receptionist's smile, is it so hard to believe that we can reprogram our days with a single word, "Super!"

When you appreciate that on a Super day you will satisfy more patients, make more sales, keep staff happier, and receive carloads of benefits to yourself in increased income, greater job security, and happier workings of your body's physiology—then you will opt for a Super day. That's because you know a Super day will bring you abundant benefits and abundant pleasure.

We select our priorities on the basis of whatever we believe will bring us the greatest benefits.

Could any dentist seriously doubt the benefits of programming a Super day? Surely not after he has treated his dozenth case of psychosomatic toothache. If we know that people can program illness, then why should it be difficult to believe we can also program health and happiness and wealth and success and love and whatever you want?

What the mind can conceive the body can deliver. Have a Super day!

If you decide not to, of course, that's your prerogative. You may shortcircuit the whole process with guilt, anxiety, worry, stress, jealousy, rage, sorrow, loneliness, discouragement, depression, or rejection. But why? None of the above are any fun. And all will succumb to a firm positive program designed to create their opposites.

Negatives turn "I will" into "I might." And "I might" simply doesn't work. It would be like running a computer on half its required current. It doesn't work half as well. It plainly doesn't work at all.

Your car won't run on half gas and half water. Nobody gets half a date, half a sale, or half a touchdown. There is no part-time employment for our programs.

We need only one person's permission to fail! Ourselves.

Dr. Frank learned that the hard way. He needed a washer for a piece of equipment in his lab. He ordered it from his supplier and waited. And he waited and waited. The longer he waited, the madder he got. He fussed and fumed to his salesman. He complained to his staff and patients. When he took it home to complain about it there, his wife said, "Why don't you go buy the washer at a hardware store?"

Dr. Frank did. In three minutes he had replaced the 16¢ washer. And then he realized what had happened to him. He had allowed a 16¢ washer to reprogram his attitude for weeks—a washer that took him three minutes to replace.

Have you ever let a 16¢ washer reprogram your days? Most of us have. But what a waste. In retrospect, Dr. Frank laughs about the incident. He learned a valuable lesson that he frequently tells on himself.

Some of Dr. Bill's patients try to program him to the grumpy day they are having. He told me about one patient who recently ranted profanely about his problems. Dr. Bill quickly told him, "Sir, you have two choices. Clean up your language or take your business to someone who will tolerate such behavior." The patient apologized, became a pussycat, and Dr. Bill's Super! day continued.

He told me about another patient who always comes stalking to the dental chair bearing an envelope or a piece of a grocery sack in hand. On it are listed a multitude of complaints. She doesn't want to miss a single opportunity to lay her negative programs on him.

"How do you handle it, Bill?" I asked. "Get rid of her?"

"I wouldn't let her leave my practice for the world. She's an important teaching aid on my schedule," he said.

"Teaching aid? How so?"

"I turn her frowns into smiles in a matter of minutes. I show my staff how we program our patients to our programs, not theirs. No, Marge is just too valuable for us to let go."

Another colleague programs his staff when they start working for him. It's pretty nifty, so I stole it from him. His introductory talk goes like this:

> There are three people you have to please on this job, and I am *not* one of them. [Huh?] That's right, I'm not one of them.
>
> One of them is the customers. They pay our bills, pay your salary and mine, and make everything happen. We will do everything reasonable to please them.
>
> Another is the staff. We have a carefully selected, superb staff working here. They feel it is a privilege to be here, just as I feel it is to have them. I will allow no one to be a seed of dissension on our fine team.
>
> The third person you must please is yourself. You have to feel you are growing, making a useful contribution to the community, and are being fairly rewarded for your efforts.
>
> Now, if you please the customers, get along with the rest of the staff, and satisfy yourself, there is no way you could fail to please me.

At the outset, his employees understand his program for them. He has handed them a script of the role he wants them to play. That script will contribute to an improvement in his lifestyle.

People who attempt to program you today must compete with your past, which has programmed your present and clouded your future. "Revenge is mine," said the Lord. Good arrangement. I don't have time, energy, or room for it. Nobody else does either.

Booker T. Washington said, "I will permit no man to narrow or degrade my soul by making me hate him." No one can make you feel inferior without your permission. Don't give that permission, for you are inferior to no one!

These minor, homely, emotional elements separate winners from losers—not the major elements. How you address the elevator operator or cabbie probably contributes more to your success than you believed possible. Even our choice of words has an impact on those with whom we share them.

A young boy was being prepared for his first date by his mother. She promised him all would go well if he would remember to give his date a compliment. As the evening wore on, he tried and tried to think of a compliment to give. Finally, a thought occurred and he said, "You sure don't sweat much for a fat person."

"I sure like your odor, lady," and "I love your fragrance, my dear," both mean approximately the same thing. But it's not difficult to guess which statement will produce more favorable results.

With a PASSION! program for yourself and for those around you, you can achieve the wildest dream you have ever entertained. There are two ifs: (1) *If* you have the dream and (2) *If* you have the passion to make it happen.

It starts with SUPER! Have a super day.

SECTION II:

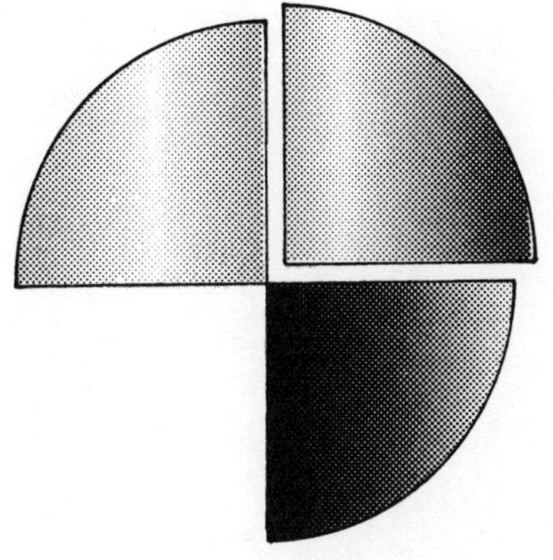

Coming Down from the Mountaintop

6
SOCK IT TO YOURSELF

The lead dog is the only one with a change of view.

—Eskimo proverb

So far we've shown the benefits of programming the most beautiful and powerful computer in the world: your mind. You simply tell it what you want, and the results will occur, guaranteed by The Maker of all minds. It's exactly that simple.

Once you program your mind to produce benefits, you carry it out in three steps:

1. Learn the rules
2. Take a risk
3. Go after your goals with PASSION!

We start now. The following questions need your answers. Take a bold, felt-tipped pen. Fill in the blanks. Be sure to think big.

That's as in BIG. Go just past the realm of what you reasonably could be expected to achieve in the next twelve months.

You must think big for the same reason that you wouldn't program your personal computer—the machine, not the mind—to calculate change for a dollar. There is no need to place a thumbtack with a sledge hammer. To use your very personal computer—your mind, not the machine—to produce a box of chocolate chip cookies, when it could just as well produce a corner on the cocoa bean market, would be a serious waste of talent.

Many people still balk at big. They see no rational way that their mind computer can produce a result beyond that which their limited imagination can conceive. That's a shame.

Consider the most successful person you know of. You have the exact same mental computer capacity that he/she has/had. Exactly!

The easy out is to cop-out. "Well, I couldn't be *that* successful because _________." The blank is filled in with everything but the truth.

And the truth is, no one in the world has a better success mechanism than you and I do. Better used perhaps, but not better. Using ours better is what this book is all about.

So, Think BIG.

My New Year's Expectations

Twelve months from today will be ______, 19__. By then I will achieve these goals, bar none.

Here is how I want others to look on me:

____

____

____

Here are the material possessions I expect:

____

____

____

Here is where I expect to be in my job:

____

____

____

Here are the personal changes I expect in myself:

____

____

____

Here are the special relationships I want with people:

____

____

____

I assume you did not list basic food, clothing, shelter needs on these expectations. Having not listed those three essentials, there is an observation to be made.

Every expectation listed was an emotional need, rather than a logical need. Nothing wrong with that. We have already cited that we are emotional beings, with copious emotional needs far and above our logical needs.

It is the logic in us that fights against us when we find we expect more out of life than minimal successes. Our emotional selves don't deal in logic and therefore everything is possible.

Your list of expectations is very personal, very private. Store it in your *sock* drawer, so you will see it each day when you go for fresh socks. Read and reread it often, the more often the better. Each rereading creates a new reprogramming.

And the more you reprogram yourself, the more you will overcome your logical resistance to accept startling results of achievement. Your expectations never looked so good.

"Sock" it to yourself.

7
THE FIRST STEP IS THE HARDEST

If something is worth doing at all, it is worth doing well.

—*Art Schmidt*

Let's put PASSION! to work. Let's go to the office with it and look around at those four walls that trap a third of our lives.

Enriching our lives is our expectation. Just what is it within these walls that can be enriched with PASSION!? Plenty.

We cannot print (or hope to sell) a book three feet thick, so we do not have the space to walk through every application of PASSION! Obviously, beginners and retired persons have different emotional needs and applications. And there are hosts of other differences among us, not the least of which are those that result from our sex.

So let us use the professional office as the common ground for our examination of PASSION! Since all private professional offices have scores of similarities, my colleagues in nondental disciplines will realize that most of us scratch the same itch. While my itch is a dental office, it is hardly different from the scene faced daily by a physician, optometrist, veterinarian, podiatrist, or chiropractor.

While we health professionals have different initials after our names, we have far more similarities than dissimilarities. Every professional health practitioner, for example, has to deal with the same basic dozen or so practical, everyday concerns. In that regard, we water at the same trough.

CONSIDER:

1. We deal with long years of preparatory education
2. That education is weighed 95% on science and 5% on communications skills (if that much)
3. Our patients select to use our services 95% based upon communications skills and 5% on scientific assessments; they are unqualified to do otherwise
4. We face an acknowledged doctor-supply glut
5. High start-up costs cause initial practice stress
6. We must deal with myriad problems created by the personnel we employ
7. We deal with collection problems and payment problems—in part, created by the necessity of delivering service in emergency predicaments
8. We have recall problems in delivering both continuity of service as well as maintaining a preventive posture
9. Caught in a legal miasma, we face potentially crippling lawsuits that may alter sensible care into overtreatment
10. In the changing ethics/advertising vortex, we find ourselves in tricky currents that lead to conflicts with the ethics that had originated in simpler times
11. Broken and cancelled appointments waste an unfair portion of our productive time
12. Seeking quality continuing education is an ongoing challenge

13. Dealing with the influx of third-party payment systems has created new dimensions to professional practice

14. Retail health-care delivery systems have created new concerns for "busyness" in the health-care business

15. Patients' misconceptions of doctors are continuing cause for concern

16. And by no means finally, but surely included, is the fact that our best health-care delivery cannot undo what people will not do for themselves!

Indeed, there is a broad base of similarities among doctors. Health-care colleagues in different disciplines should have little difficulty transposing PASSION! into their field. The challenges are the same.

Let's put PASSION! to work. Until now we've been talking about building a head of steam. Let's employ that steam on the job and see how it can produce benefits.

A sign in a corporate boardroom sums up about all we need to know about the business of health-care delivery—and any other business for that matter:

Nothing Happens Until a Sale Is Made

If the words "business" and "sale" in that paragraph bother you, welcome to the 1980s. Hundreds (yes, hundreds) of doctors have declared bankruptcy in the past few years. No need to tell them that professional practice is a business ruled by the same business laws that rule the business world.

Since honesty is the first rule of selling, I must say to you that the terms "practice management," "patient motivation," and "patient education" are frequently used dishonestly. What we really mean when we say them is: How can I *sell* more of my services? A reasonable and honest question for any doctor who recognizes he must *sell* his services to stay in *business*. There are those two trigger words again.

Few problems plaguing any professional businessman—and, yes, all businessmen—cannot be cured by more sales. As a friend of mine says, "Give me the business volume, and I'll figure out a way to make a profit!"

There is another major element to creating a profit in health care. And that has to do with investment in the business itself. We'll examine these two elements—sales and investment in the practice—and many others as we proceed. But first, let's address the topic of more sales.

8
PROGRAM YOUR OFFICE WITH PASSION!

In the land of the blind, the one-eyed man is King.

—Anon.

Some years ago an article appeared in a journal written by a doctor who had taken over a practice left by another doctor's untimely death. His comment about the office decor was insightful, "It was an abhorrent decor to walk into. I believe he had died years before he did, and just spent the last few years of his life living in this casket he called an office."

If you are going to spend one-third of your waking life in an office, why shouldn't it be nice enough to enjoy, nice enough to keep staff happy, and nice enough to attract patients?

Do you believe that sales environments are casually produced? Cough, gasp, wheeze. Of course, they are not. But office appearance is the very first impression we offer to our patients.

It's sad how many of these first impressions have been created by well-meaning, but ill-informed family members.

Let your spouse decorate your house and a professional decorate your professional environment.

And how does that fit with PASSION!? Only in that we each must compete in the marketplace with the best we have to offer. Unless we have programmed our office environment to the max, we cannot expect results to the max. The first program, therefore, occurs in our office environment.

Consider plants: More sales occur in offices replete with copious greenery. Period.

Consider lighting: More sales occur in offices with skillful lighting. And employees stay healthier under fluorescent lights that emit 98% of the sun's spectrum. Tooth shades are picked more accurately, too.

You must consider gestalt. What is gestalt? It's simply an element of psychology stating that an impression, when delivered positively in each of the sensory modalities, becomes more than the sum of its parts. In terms of gestalt, two plus two equals five—a handsome arrangement.

The programming of our offices begins with you saying: "I will provide a selling environment." You then:

1. Learn the rules. If this means employing those who know those rules, so be it.
2. Take a chance. It may seem the height of folly to spend hundreds or thousands of dollars to create a selling environment. But a return can never be realized on an investment that never occurred.
3. Carry out your plan with PASSION! See it through now, not in some vaguely distant future time.

Question every aspect of your environment—its look, its smell, its feel.

Appropriate stereo background music, soft and selling color coordinations, a welcoming cup of coffee or tea, fresh and protected magazines, greenery, lighting, odor and noise control—these and other accents and considerations can produce an office tuned to staff enjoyment.

What happens when your staff is surrounded with a pleasurable ambience? Attitudes improve, better spirits prevail, enthusiasm for tasks elevates, and staff members fully understand the extent of your commitment to your program.

You program your staff with an elegant selling climate, which in turn begins the programming of your patients. Do you recall our visit about first impressions?

Your office is an extension of *your* personality. It reflects you as a caring professional committed to excellence—an organized, thoughtful, and sensitive human being. Patients who enter this kind of atmosphere become relaxed and preconditioned to accept your advice. Their program begins with the first contact with your office—usually by telephone. It is expanded by that fateful first view of your reception area. And it is reinforced by your staff's attitudes toward your patients.

A million-dollar practice cannot occur in a shabby environment—not by any stretch of a penny-pincher's imagination.

Decor within our office walls is the first place to begin our programming. Our staff is next. Whoops!

It almost slipped by—A Million-Dollar Practice! That's not only what I said, that's what I meant. One Million Dollars—per year—from professional health-care practice. It's totally within the reach of every health-care professional in the business of selling health-care services—One Million Dollars!

It never comes from working harder—just from working smarter.

In the 1940s and 50s every professional on the block panted after the $100,000 practice. That was the biggie reserved for select doctors. Inflation and technology have changed all that.

If you only did $100,000 last year, you were in the minor leagues, not among the elite. The elite have the secret of programming down to a science. They may not call it PASSION! per se, but they instinctively know how it works and use it as easily as you and I breathe.

Just the thought of producing one million dollars of health-care benefits in one year scares many doctors. Out of the chute it sounds greedy. Is it? If IBM increases its sales a billion dollars, is that greedy?

Most would agree it is not. They would rationalize that IBM has provided more goods and services to help other businesses, that IBM has made a useful and viable contribution to the business community and thus to the nation's welfare. IBM would, of course, pay more taxes on increased sales.

How does this differ, except on scale, with an individual entrepreneur whether he sells insurance policies or health care?

Surely there is need for expansion of our services, despite what seems to be a doctor glut. I believe the supposed doctor glut is a misstatement of fact. The problem is not too many doctors; it is too few users of doctors' services. There is a shortage of patients.

Experts tell me the same is true for optometrists, podiatrists, and all other health-care disciplines. There is an enormous *need* for services. (See chapter 11 on advertising.) Meeting that need must be a *noblesse oblige* of doctors of every stripe. But there is also an enormous lack of *want*.

When you have actually trod the path from practice commencement to the million-dollar level, you learn an amazing thing. It takes little more effort, and in many respects less, to run a million-dollar practice than it does a two, three, or four hundred-thousand-dollar practice.

It takes no more real effort *if* you have programmed your office, your staff, your patients, and most of all yourself to make it happen. Once those programs are operable, startling things begin to occur.

You will serve more people, to be sure. But you will not sacrifice the quality of the service if you have structured sound operating programs into your plan. You will employ more people, use more goods, and use more support services and supplies. And you will enjoy a better return on your investment of blood, sweat, and fears.

And you will pay more taxes.

9
PROGRAM YOUR STAFF WITH PASSION!

No one ever loses when he surrounds himself with winners.

—DAS

To attract quality staff away from factory production lines, you must create a package of benefits that competes. Gone are the days when it was such a privilege to work for a doctor that he could hire for a pittance and treat like a hireling those who helped him earn his scampi.

Today's staff doesn't care how much you know until they know how much you care. You show that in countless ways: how your treat them in front of patients; how you compensate them for extra effort; how you motivate continuing performance; how you train them for growth in the field; what responsibilities you give them; the climate within the office; how you correct their deficiencies and gaffes; how you back them in patient confrontations; how you communicate with them day by day; and how much you truly care about their fulfillment in this effort upon which you are all embarked.

Together these elements program your staff to complement your productivity, to be a plus and change the odds. What are the odds? A Rockefeller study produced these dramatic numbers telling why patients leave you—or why customers leave other businesses:

1% die
3% move away
5% leave for other friendships
9% leave for competitive reasons
14% leave due to product dissatisfaction
68% leave *because of an attitude of indifference* toward the patient by an employee

With strong employee programming, we can change those odds in our favor. It is, after all, easier to keep an existing customer—and more profitable—than it is to seek his replacement. For that matter it is less expensive to keep existing staff than it is to seek their replacement.

When my practice was in a building housing several professional offices, my neighbor came into my office one day and sighed, "Well, I finally got rid of her!"

"Who, Bob?"

"My receptionist, thank God."

"Trouble?"

"Big trouble. She was curt with patients. She never took emergencies if it made us work a little harder. On her bowling night nobody was ever seen late. She didn't call to confirm appointments ahead of time, and she was lousy on financial arrangements and collections. Whew!"

"Gee, that's too bad. How long was she with you?"

"Six years."

SIX YEARS! Putting up with that sort of performance for six years is mind-boggling. If your staff refuses your programs, cut them from your life at once. It's hard enough doing our job when all our shoulders are heaving in the same traces. It's impossible when anyone fails to accept your programs.

Sixty-eight percent of our patients leave us *because of an attitude of indifference!* Can you afford that loss? Of course not. No one can stay alive in today's keen, competitive climate with losses like that.

Once we have programmed ourselves in what I call "The Toughest Sale in the World," have programmed our office to become a selling environment, and have programmed our staff to work in this single-minded direction, we will have created a sales atmosphere—an atmosphere that can thrive in the rough and tumble world of professional competition.

10
PROGRAM YOUR SIZE WITH PASSION!

When elephants fight, it's the ants that get hurt.

—African proverb

When these programs begin to interact, growth *will* occur. A patient base will be retained with better statistics than those of the Rockefeller study. Those patients will be more receptive to your suggestions for both corrective and preventive health maintenance. And they will be a more proficient referral source.

New patients will be attracted to the environment you have created, and growth with occur. How will you handle it? Your answer is crucial to the longevity of those practice principles you espouse. First, let's again talk about **big.** Is it good to grow **that** big?

In the middle of the 1970s, I opened my dental practice with a hangover. No, not the kind caused by alcohol, but a more insidious kind—a hangover of trite dental aphorisms that had been laid on me by those who had taught me the profession. Perhaps you have heard, or harbored, some of these, too:

Big is bad.
Small is good.
Expensive is best.
Cheap is worst.
Get busy, then expand.
Nice dentists don't advertise.
Dental insurance will wreck dentistry.

These were as logical as "white is pure" and "black is evil." I don't fault those who taught me, for there is an element of truth in every fable. But having discovered the power of PASSION! and wanting to see what it could do in dentistry, I had to first cope with the "what ifs" I believed could happen.

What if dental insurance took America's industrial complex by storm? What if the freshly minted Bates Supreme Court decision allowed not only lawyers to advertise but dentists, too? What if I got too busy before I expanded and couldn't handle the new business? What if I tried to be truly cost-competitive in fees? What if I did these things and grew to a size that I could barely dream of?

If I had been younger than midforties, I might have bought those old maxims at face value. I would at least have more time remaining to do things differently later. But, being an impatient sort and seeing the handwriting in the *Wall (Street Journal)*, I opted to go for it, chuck those chestnuts, and take a chance that they were wrong.

I already knew the rules (step one). I now was willing to take a chance and risk failure (step two). All that remained was to practice with PASSION!

From the opening gun, it took 28 months to reach that first million dollars of production, less time for the second million, and so on. Along the way some eye-openers occurred in terms of economy of size.

Economy of Size

If the overhead for a five-day, 8-to-5 office is 60% of production, opening for extra hours each week will not eat 60% of the increased production. Add a noon hour, add 5–8 p.m. daily, add some afternoons normally closed and a few Saturday hours, and you'll find the additional overhead for those hours will more closely approach 40%. That's an increased gross profit margin of 20%—a number that would excite the interest of any businessman.

Marketing programs need to be more vigorous for a larger operation than for a small operation. Marketing costs, however, when spread over a larger production volume become proportionately smaller. For example, an office might spend $4,000 annually for a display ad in the Yellow Pages. This would be 4% for a $100,000 practice, but only 0.4% of a $1,000,000 practice—both ads accomplishing the same goal.

Bigness also creates buying power. Often, suppliers give preferred customer discounts to sell to larger offices. And, too, larger offices can use volume buying to achieve even greater savings.

Broaden Patient Base

Many years ago a colleague who was my mentor cautioned me to never pressure a patient to follow my recommendations for his health care. A patient who is sold softly is led into a buying posture, he counseled. A patient who is sold hard is pushed into a sale and will ultimately reject the position in which he has been placed, my colleague added.

He likened it to moving a piece of string from here to there. "You can push it or you can pull it, but only one of those ways works!" I later heard that General Eisenhower had used the same illustration during the days of his European offensive. It worked both for him and for my mentor on me.

The advice has been useful. Those patients who give us the most frequent headaches are those we have pushed rather than led. A broad patient base eases the pressure of having to sell. Thus, we are afforded the luxury of selling our patients softly.

A large operation, by its very nature, will attract a greater influx of new patients. A broad patient base provides greater opportunities for continuing referrals in that larger circles of influence are at work.

Recent recessionary times have pointed out the immense value to an ongoing operation of a large patient base.

Convenience

The number one attraction to patients has repeatedly been shown to be convenience. Convenience in location usually means a location with a high traffic count. It's a location where people are and can get to easily. But locations sporting high traffic cost more. This cost percentage is reduced, however, when laid against a larger gross.

Convenience means offering expanded hours for those who cannot avail themselves of the usual eight to five.

Convenience means offering the services of another in-house doctor when you cannot fulfill all the patients' wants.

Convenience in a multiple-doctor office allows 24-hour emergency duties to be spread over several doctors rather than being borne by one.

Convenience means an increased ability to see emergency patients as promptly as they wish to be seen.

Convenience is a number one asset of a larger operation and a number one attraction for new patients.

Administrivia

Some colleagues have offered the observation that administration of a large operation "Must be a nightmare! And especially when you have to deal with a couple dozen women employees!" That comment is highly sexist and personally is quite offensive to me. Dealing with a dozen employees of *any* stripe can geometrically increase an employer's problems. This question implies difficulty because the employee is a women. Not true.

In our practice we have so few problems among staff that I marvel at their compatibility. In large measure I attribute this to a willingness to rid ourselves of problems once we have identified them. A "problem" in this instance being an employee who is unwilling to become a member of our "team."

Hearsay evidence, stemming from scores of practitioners with whom I have visited across this land, supports the thesis that doctors are afraid to rid themselves of poorly functioning, unproductive staff. The reduction that accrues to them in income and—perhaps more importantly—in joy of practicing their profession must be one of the plagues of the profession in America today.

There is an old phrase I once learned as a children's dentist: More dentists are afraid of children than children of dentists. Paraphrase this to read: More dentists are afraid of staff than staff of dentists. I tell this to dentists who pose that ill-phrased remark.

I also point out to them that they probably spend more time administering a small practice than they would a large one. In our practice there are several reasons for such efficiencies. First, we have a thorough set of office policies. We have to. Each employee must know how to respond to various situations. And they must know the office position on myriad details that might come up. This reduces much of the normal administrivia.

Second, we have training manuals that, along with cooperative senior employees, help new staff members get in tune with our programs more quickly.

Third, outside interferences from sales personnel are screened by staff. For example, if a salesman calls to present a product or program, a staff member—the one who most often deals with those particular matters—goes over the salesman's proposal. If she believes it is worthy of our attention, she gives me a capsule summary and we see if we want to explore it. If we do, she sits in on the sales visit and gives me input to help us make a better decision.

Staff Expansion

A large staff is an advantage in numerous ways. Specialization may occur so that one employee handles all insurance matters, another collections, another recalls, another sterilization and tray setups. Another is responsible for X-ray maintenance, another does all supply ordering and so on.

In this manner each employee is in charge of a smaller piece of the operation. Therefore, a higher level of performance can be expected. This reduces performance loss when an employee is on vacation or ill.

Being large allows us to have our own technicians in our own laboratory. Thus, we can offer our patients quick denture repair and in-house laboratory consultations on difficult cases. These are superb conveniences for the patients.

Doctor Benefits

Because of a large, well-trained staff, doctors work more relaxed and the work is more fun. With overhead spread over the production of several producers, it becomes a shared burden of less magnitude. In a large office, doctors may work less and, because they're working with less pressure, may actually sell and produce more.

Patients benefit because a doctor is always available to treat emergencies, even when the rest of the doctor staff is on vacation. Doctors may easily consult with one another on stickler cases. Doctors may subspecialize in areas of greater interest. And they may improve office services by taking a variety of continuing education courses and then sharing their new knowledge with the other doctors.

Disadvantages of Bigness

A potential for services to be delivered impersonally exists in every practice, but no more or less in a large operation. It is something that requires a great deal of self-discipline to conquer in any health-care circumstance.

Rapid growth may cause cash flow problems of no small magnitude. This, too, demands rigid self-discipline so that the office doesn't run away with the practice.

When my daughters were toddlers, I worried about many things that might happen to them as they grew up. But, as the years rolled by, I made a discovery most parents make. Most of the things I worried about never happened. And many others, when they did occur, could be dealt with because we had learned along the way—we were older and maybe a little bit wiser. We had grown with our children just as a doctor grows with his practice.

Big is neither more nor less likely to be bad. It doesn't turn on the size of the practice. The determinant is the stature of the practitioners—the same thing it's always been.

I cited the cost of a Yellow Pages ad. There is a lot of feeling about this in dentistry and other professions. Let's look at advertising for a moment.

11
PROGRAM YOURSELF TO MARKET

Why is it that a doctor can sleep in advertised pajamas on an advertised mattress, awake to an advertised alarm clock, drink advertised orange juice and eat advertised toast, drive to the office in his advertised car, and work with advertised equipment—and say: I don't believe in advertising!? Then, when he dies, his widow advertises his practice for sale.

Dentists advertise—in Rotary and Lions clubs, on school boards, everywhere. They promote themselves as Dr. Nice Guy in hopes of garnering more business and attracting patients. Countless stock portfolios and mink coats have been gained by such carefully planned activities as seeking the presidency of Jaycees, chairing Children's Dental Health programs, or stumping for popular causes.

And yet, mention advertising and dentistry in the same breath to many of these dentists, and they recoil in horror.

"Advertise in dentistry?" they gasp. "It will ruin professionalism. The dignity of the profession will go down the drain. People will choose their dentist for all the wrong reasons. Dentistry will cost more and you can kiss quality goodbye. Advertise in dentistry? Never!"

Dental advertising's never-never land just got here. The Supreme Court says we can. The Federal Trade Commission says we should. Will dour predictions for the future of our profession now come true? Probably not.

Fighting a change in the dental-care delivery system insinuates the system is working well. If you believe that, you believe in the Tooth Fairy.

Half the citizenry of the United States did not see a dentist last year. It's a national disgrace. Of the half who sought dental care, half of them doctor-shopped during the year. If people are so content with what we deliver now, why do they shop around so much? Sixty-four percent of our population of 209 million persons have unmet dental needs. That's enough to book our entire dental-care system solid, forever!

Yet "busyness" seminars continue as we meet to figure out why the only time most people open their mouths to us is to yawn. Marketing conferences pack dentists in to teach them about the dawning of retail dentistry. Collectively, we use cutesy ad campaigns that "Sparkle, Glow, Beam, and Dazzle" us—but not our patients. If this is good, how bad can bad be?

The Chosen Few

Today, there is no intelligent way to choose a dentist. To say that advertising may mislead people into choosing their dentist unwisely is to imply that people choose wisely now. Nothing could be further from the truth. People choose their dentist emotionally, not intellectually. Currently, people choose their dentist for all the wrong reasons. They have no other choice.

Your new patient may come to you because you are conveniently located, have a smart office, keep long hours, accept Mastercard and Visa, have a sweetheart staff, employ happy gas, offer free parking, or have a name beginning with an A at the top of the Yellow Pages listings. None of those reasons are logical. They are all emotional.

The same is true if your patients chose you because of your long years in practice. Some dentists have twenty years of experience, while others have one year of experience twenty times over. If you were chosen because you do quality work, how was that quality evaluated? Probably by a person who wouldn't know a margin from margarine. Again, it was an emotional bias, not an intellectual choice.

The American Dental Association booklet, *How to Be a Wise Dental Consumer,* is an example. It suggests several ways to choose a dentist, the first of which is "Ask your friends, neighbors and co-workers." What, pray tell, do friends and neighbors know about choosing a dentist wisely? A dart board would be faster and just as logical.

"Ask a faculty member of a dental school." The odds are he doesn't know the market any better than the local third-grade teacher. He may know a few officers of dental societies, but being a dental officer guarantees nothing but a lot of thankless work. He may know some former students but won't know if any growth occurred after dental school. Also, he will not know dentists who have entered his market area from other schools. Some of those imported dentists *actually* do quality work.

"Check with a hospital having an accredited dental service." How a hospital dentist is blessed with powers to evaluate community dentistry escapes me.

"Check the ADA directory." Now we're getting down to the meat. In the directory you learn the year a dentist graduated, his school, and his zip code. This should help the layman, if he is into Chinese astrology. (A person born in the year of the Goat might not want to be attended by a dentist who graduated in the year of the Rooster.) If the eager patient is into numerology, he can attach a meaning to the ADA number listed for dentists in his area. Otherwise, the ADA directory is as useful a tool in choosing a dentist as the license plate on a doctor's car.

"Check with your family physician (ask who provides his care)." Most physicians don't know an inlay from an onlay. Why should they? Physicians, too, rate their dentists on emotional factors. "Check with your pharmacist" has the same effect. Our choices of physicians and pharmacists are made the same way—emotionally.

Various public interest groups have kicked up a flurry of amalgam dust by publishing directories of dentists. Those directories reveal hard data on topics such as education, equipment, payment plans, office hours, and disciplines of special interest to the dentist. These publishing efforts have been met with dentists' emotions ranging from indignation to rage. In the absence of a better method, perhaps it would be wise for dentists to take the initiative and publish a meaningful body of data that would beat the ask-your-buddy system.

We want to think our patients choose us for all the right reasons. They do not. There is little likelihood they ever will because buying decisions are emotional decisions, born apart from logic. Our patients choose us, not on the basis of the superb quality of service we render—since none of them is qualified to judge that quality—but on the basis of every emotional factor under the operatory light.

There is just as much opportunity to mislead your friends in the church choir, to mislead the community because you are the newly announced president of your dental society, or to mislead everyone who has heard you took a dozen Boy Scouts to a Jamboree, as there is to mislead the public in a full-page newspaper advertisement. Really, what is the difference?

Dig Our Dignity

The stated difference is in the deterioration of professional dignity, which some dentists feel occurs through advertisement. Personally, I do not feel I've lost any professional dignity because national TV exposed a dentist Superman dressed like a clown. (Or was it the other way around?) Neither does my dignity suffer when dentists shoot themselves, get drunk, or fill hyenas' teeth.

The point is there is no such thing as the dignity of the profession. There is only the professional dignity of individual dentists. Each of us builds or wrecks our own. The public fully understands that. People do not ask the profession to protect their dental health. They ask one specific dentist. We should understand it, too, even if Dr. Big Ads hypes the whole community on how great he is.

If Dr. Slippery cannot deliver quality dental care, the public will find him out faster when he advertises. My guarantee to you is this: *Please a patient and he may tell his friends; displease him and he will tell the world.*

If you want to fret over professional deterioration, here's a handful to keep your fretter working overtime. What about dentists who judge another's work with a raised eyebrow or a tongue cluck, followed by a grunt and a shake of the head? It's probably overdramatization to throw your head in your hands and cry out: "Dr. Schmidt actually did this work for you? Oh my gosh! I thought he was through with that sort of thing!"

How often do colleagues chop each other up like liver paté? Plenty! You know that is true because it always comes back. But mudthrowers lose ground when they sling. In such cases the dentist is saying that the patient was stupid enough to buy bad dentistry. He doesn't just put down the former dentist; he puts down the patient as well.

What about half the dentists in America who refuse to treat 21 million welfare recipients? Could you imagine, in your wildest imaginings, a circumstance that reflects more poorly on the state of the art in dental America? Hardly.

Or how about profiteering? There is no reason in the world for a denture to cost a patient's life savings, plus a loan from Junior. But it often does. And this very profiteering has paved asphalt streets with gold for denturists.

Another advertising windmill that is getting a lot of tilting action is cost. This really is grasping at straws. Dentistry is not higher quality because or when it costs more.

What about dentists who aren't dealing with a full deck? With all the professional chatter about stress in dentistry, there must be a host of overstressed fingers plying the dental business out there in Stressville, USA. What is their effect on the dignity of the profession?

How about dentists who wish they had not entered the drill mill, who refuse to nudge their sons and daughters into dentistry, and who are bored to tears with the means of their livelihood? How well do these doctors represent the dignity of dentistry?

What about dentists who attempt to practice without hugging continual education to their bosom? Even in states requiring annual CE quotas, how many quotas are filled by a half-hour spin through aisles of shiny gadgets at dental conventions?

There are, indeed, ways to deteriorate our group dignity. But we do them one by one, one on one, not collectively.

Dentistry often costs what it does in America because of inefficient practices that multiply patient costs. We are today at the same threshold we were 25 years ago when we passed from solo, standup operatories with single assistants to multiple, sitdown operatories with four- and now six-handed dentistry.

Abundant evidence in the business world demonstrates that costs decrease when advertising introduces a product or a service. For example, think of ball-point pens, calculators, and razor blades. The Supreme Court noted this in its Bates decision brief. They called attention to evidence that advertising has contributed to lowering the cost of eyeglasses, prescription drugs, and legal services.

If it is true that half of our patients doctor-shopped last year, at least one reason they did so was cost. Other reasons were convenience and a failure on the part of their current dentist to communicate with them. Talking *to* our patients does not supplant talking *with* our patients.

In the U.S., it's reported that more dental supplies are purchased from discount, mail-order suppliers than from local suppliers by doctors who, themselves, decry discounters. Is there a message there?

Doctors who drive all over town to save a buck on hunting boots, case beer, and megavitamins find it difficult to understand that the public does the same thing.

The Supreme Court, noting the objection about advertising in dentistry raising its costs, pointed out that such an idea presumes the public is unaware that dentists earn a living from dentistry. Few people, the Court added, climb in a dental chair expecting free service.

What we can do in advertising is to do exactly what the word means: to announce. This must be honest and stripped of hyperbole.

Advertising without hype informs. It tells of availability of service, kinds of services offered, who the doctors are behind an office name, payment plans available, and the like. In short, these announcements help people make decisions based more on data than on the emotionalism of word of mouth.

Decisions based on data may still be wrong decisions. But decisions based on hearsay have far greater chance to be in error. How any dental organization can recommend hearsay referrals as a "wise" course of action escapes me.

Where is advertising in dentistry leading us? Well, it doesn't necessarily contribute to the deterioration of our dignity. We do enough things, individually, to so do without any help from "Eight Old Men and One Woman" and the FTC. It does not contribute to choosing a dentist more emotionally because that's the way patients choose us now.

Advertising will not lead to a poorer quality of service any more than does greed. And dental services will not cost more than they do now because of advertising. Dr. Slick will never steal *our* patients whom we are satisfying with convenience, quality service, good communication, and fair fees.

If we don't let our high-speed handpieces blow away our cool and if we keep our paranoia in check, perhaps advertising in dentistry may let a little of the dark leak out of our operatories. Maybe we can entice a few of those hundreds of millions of nonbelievers into taking better care of themselves, as can only happen in a dental office.

Nice dentists *can* advertise—with dignity. And when it is done skillfully, no one even knows that you advertise. I will venture that no more than a handful of our patient base, which numbers well into five digits, even suspects that we advertise.

We do. But we do so with dignity, finesse, and a rifle aimed toward our markets—not a shotgun aimed at the community.

12 MARKET WITH PASSION!

You cannot get pinned when you are on top.

—Old wrestling expression

Quick: How many new patients did you invite into your practice last month? This year to date? Last year? Do you know all three of those numbers? Super! Most of your colleagues don't.

Exactly what current efforts of yours produce new patients? Do you know that, too? That rates still another Super! Few professionals bother to learn these vital statistics. "Vital" is precisely the right word. Life and death of a professional's practice are what we're talking about.

There's one more question: What is it you want your marketing to do for you? Yes, I know: Get more business. But how? What kind of new business?

If you answered "new patients" to the last question that's good, but you missed what I call The Hidden Goldmine in any practice. We'll get to that in short order, but first let's go back to our vital statistics. They are simple to accumulate: "Mary, when each new patient enters our practice, enter that info on a chart. List the referral sources as these:

1. Friends
2. Family
3. Staff
4. Newspaper
5. Yellow Pages
6. Other (be specific)

"Then put them on my desk the first of each month."

You have now programmed Mary and will never again be blank when asked where your patients originated. Of course, add "Please" and "Thank you" to Mary's program.

Reading these statistics each month—and recording the grand totals on a chart of some sort—gives you a measure of where you are. Watching new numbers lay against the old gives you a measure of where you are going and where you have been. Nice information to have, especially if you are going to do any new marketing. How could you otherwise assess results?

Until we know these basics, we have no business going anywhere with our marketing. And that's because that is precisely where our business will go—nowhere.

Where can we go for new patients? There are several specific markets:

1. The *newcomer,* which also includes oldcomers who have no dentist ties
2. The *emergency patient*
3. *Satisfied patients* who already have happy dental ties
4. The *silver platter* patient

"Silver platter" patients are those patients other dentists hand to you. They have lost contact with a former dentist, usually due to a communications breakdown, and they now seek your golden touch.

Caveat Doctor! Beware! These people, who tell you long tales of real and imagined insults by their former dentist, will likely soon turn tail on you and tell the next dentist on their hit list of the indignities suffered at your hands.

In my exuberant youth, I relished these patients and was eager to prove myself the master of their dental fates. It rarely worked out. They are the unprogrammable ones whom we divorce from our practice as soon as possible—if not sooner.

You may have every Silver Platter patient in our town. They are emotional misfits trying to create a crowd to observe their self-imposed misery. I don't want to be part of that crowd.

When a patient starts a story about a colleague, I hush him with an instant admonition: "Look we start from today. If you want my help, maybe I can and maybe not. But I don't want to hear what happened elsewhere because it won't influence how I will treat you."

Just a brief aside here for a quick reprogram of the "guilty" patient. You see them all the time, as do we. They haven't had dental service in years. They are ashamed of the mouthful of neglect they carry about.

Personally, I believe that fear of reproach from a father- or mother-figure dentist deters whole hosts of those who avoid us. If the ADA were to work on a national campaign that would really produce results, it should emphasize an attack on patient guilt, rather than such inanities as: "Decay Will Wreck Detooth!" How much do you suppose was spent developing that ad? (I was going to call it a "rotten" ad but that's too much of a play on "decay.")

Here's the sentence we impose on the guilty: "Look Betty, if you want a spanking, you'll have to go to your mother. We don't deliver spankings, just good dental service. We start from today. I'm just glad you had the good sense to get in here now. And, yes, I've seen worse, more times than you can count."

I've had patients break down and cry with relief after that amnesty I've granted them. And yet I've heard colleagues brag about how they try their victims and sentence them to many lashes with their dentist's tongue. Incredibly obtuse programming, but it happens—all the time.

We don't want the Silver Platter patient. We can't take patients who already are being well-served by my many good dentist buddies. So that only leaves the newcomer, the oldcomer who has no dentist ties, and the emergency patient. Of course, some of those emergency patients come to us because they can't find their dentist when they need him.

A couple years after this practice started, I saw that no one in town offered 24-hour answering service for general dentistry. So we did.

Yes, it is sometimes inconvenient to carry the pager always. Yes, we sometimes get ridiculous calls. Yes, we get a share of calls from druggies. But we do offer a solid service to our patients who have learned that dental emergencies don't always occur from nine to five on weekdays.

For the small cost, we make many friends by the simple expedient of being available. Strange how many dentists take vacations without a thought as to who is going to service their patient family. I recall the first patient to call me on page. He needed relief for a toothache. I provided that and later a full upper and lower denture. That call alone paid for 10 months of the page service.

When I go out with my pager, people ask: "Oh, are you a doctor?" I reply: "No, I'm not a REAL doctor, I'm a dentist, and my patients deserve my best at all hours, not just when it's convenient for me." (Little joke there on REAL doctor. You other nonphysicians probably don't have that problem like we dentists do.)

Druggies either sound whiney or have perfect diction, it seems. They often know too much about drugs or are too specific about what they "need." We counter that by prescribing antibiotics and minimal, milder pain-relievers. Then we tell the pharmacist that he/she must check an ID before dispensing *and* he cannot dispense the pain-reliever if the patient fails to purchase the antibiotic.

Fortunately, our pharmaceutical community has good tracking sources and keeps a hot list of names of strong suspects among drug abusers. We always ask them to check that list if the patient is suspect.

Back to marketing. Is that the only place to get new business? Decidedly not. New patients? Yes. New business? No.

The Hidden Gold Mine

There is a vast gold mine of untapped business that we all successfully avoid. If "The Toughest Sale in the World" is yourself, what is the "Easiest Sale in the World"? A sale to an existing customer.

He has already demonstrated his faith in you. He has already handed over some of his crisp green to you in exchange for something you've done for him. The trouble is you haven't done it all—not all he needs, at any rate.

A dentist friend once told me: "More undone dentistry walks out of dental offices than is done in them." Think about that! There's a world of wisdom in it. If you've practiced over a few months, you will probably agree—flat out.

Take it a step further. Are you seeing all the family members in every family in which you have at least one patient member? Who is? No one.

Are you seeing all the friends in the circle of influence surrounding each patient of yours? No one else is either.

Are your patients buying *all* of your advice? Is every patient following your recall advice to the letter? Yeah, me too.

That's the hidden gold mine in your practice and mine. If we could only tap 1% of it, we would be too busy to have time to read (or write) this book! It's the most beautiful opportunity in the world and hardly ever gets noticed.

Joe Girard is listed in the *Guinness Book of World Records* as the World's Greatest Salesman. Maybe he is. He says something profound when he speaks of "circles of influence." He says everyone has a circle of 250 people they can influence.

That's about 20 tons of people, which creates the value of powerful first impressions. It also creates the value of marketing to an existing patient base for new business over marketing to a new patient flow. It's easier. It's cheaper. It gets better results. And it also takes some work. But then what doesn't?

Marketing Principles

Sometimes I'm asked which marketing program of ours works best? That's like asking which vitamin in the nutritional supplement I take makes me feel best. Gosh, I don't know.

Seems like a strange answer, but it isn't. No one can assess marketing on an item basis. Yes, to be sure, there are ways to count new leads, new patients who attest it was one thing or another that caused them to go to an office—postcard or coupon response, for example. But there is only one measure of a marketing program—bottom line.

Did the company make a profit? Did it grow? That's really all that matters. Your company historian (that's your accountant) will answer that for you at year end, if not sooner.

That's one principle: *Marketing success is only assessed by how the business did this year over past years.*

Another is: *Never hunt with a shotgun if a rifle will do it better.* A large splashy ad in the local paper may create a little business. But it's a shotgun. It's not cost-effective because you are spending too many dollars reaching thousands of satisfied patients in other offices. That's a waste of dollars.

Still another marketing principle is: *Shower spray never erodes the enamel in your bathtub, but a drippy faucet will.* Big splashes are not only cost-ineffective, they don't bring results like small, repetitive notices (ads) do. Stay with it steadily to get best results. At any given moment someone needs your services. Be visible when those daily needs arise, and you will receive more benefits.

An old advertising adage goes: *If it ain't broke don't fix it!* That's another principle to learn. Advertising agents say that one of their biggest problems is that company people get tired of seeing their own advertising long before the public does. If you have a winner, ride it again and again.

Finally: *Don't expect miracles.* They never occur. You will never receive a vast influx of new business from any marketing campaign. Never. But you will get some if it is conceived and executed properly. So hang in there. Marketing works, but only when pointed in the right direction with the proper instruments and when it is assessed in its final analysis by growth of profit.

Who does the conception? You, of course. It's your business life on the line. You need to know as much as you can about marketing to make it work. But you aren't an advertising specialist. Knowing these few guidelines does not qualify you to make all the decisions.

The big important decisions? Yes. But we need skilled professionals just as they at times need our skills. Help is available both from ad agencies and from in-house talent at printers, Yellow

Pages, and specialty ad concerns. Don't worry that they don't know dentistry. They know communication.

Your first big decision is to decide how much to spend. Two to three percent of last year's gross might be a fair starting point. Then again you may wish to go larger or smaller, depending on your inclinations, needs, and personal feelings about marketing. It is strictly your choice.

Make that choice alone, not in the heat of a fantastic sales pitch by a fervent disciple of, "The ad of the century, Doctor, that you cannot do without, Doctor, because everyone is doing it, Doctor, and you don't want to be left out, Doctor, and this is the absolutely last chance to sign up and you better get aboard, Doctor, or you'll be lost, drowned, immersed by your competitors." Bull!

You decide where to spend *your* bucks. You get professionals to help you get more mileage for fewer bucks; but they're your bucks to spend, no one else's.

Two more things. First, I'll tell you some ad methods that are guaranteed to cost you big money with zero results. You would do more good to print your name and phone number on dollar bills and hand them out at the supermarket than to use these methods. Maybe you've read somewhere that someone made them work for him. I doubt it. I read somewhere that *Hustler* publisher Larry Flynt is a born-again Christian, too.

Second, I'll tell you how we address these markets and a bit of the philosophy behind our approach. We are never more right than our bottom line. Fortunately, we've been blessed in that regard. You may get better results from different methods. Surely, what we do may not work in your market, but then we only have to market in our market.

I've listed some of my marketing pratfalls. When I'm called about others like them (every day?) I tell the caller, "I'll be glad to consider it for next year's budget, but we are fully budgeted for this year. Please send materials only. If I am interested, I will call for a sales visit. I will not expect to have any more calls on this."

I have to do it that way because, if an idea is good this year, it will be just as good next year. Good ideas don't fold. They grow. Make an idea prove itself. Also, I refuse to be reprogrammed. We are programmed along solid lines of growth that we know work. I will not let those programs be deterred by others' programs.

We do not screen phone calls at our office. I am available to talk to anyone; if I cannot speak just then, I call back. So I get a lot of baloney calls. I also get the frequent pitches for charities, as all of us do. (I have to give my name just to talk to my lawyer's secretary. Egad!)

Our standard response to the charity pitch is that my staff has authority to give a few bucks to any seemingly legitimate charity out of petty cash. "Don't even tell me about it, just do it." If I'm on the phone with a fundraiser, I tell him to either stop by for a couple of bucks or send me literature on it (most have no literature) and we'll consider it for next year's gift giving.

The pratfalls of my marketing:

BOWLING SCORE SHEETS	Stupid
CHURCH BULLETINS	PTL but ridiculous!
PEN AND PENCILS	Outrageous
CITY AND ZONING MAPS	Impossible
TELEPHONE BOOK COVERS	Who looks at them?
SPECIAL NEWSPAPER SECTIONS	Our ad would get lost, like we'd be
SPECIAL EVENT PROGRAMS	Who cares
CITY GAMES	Talk about games, with my money!

There are probably others but that's a quick few. Since you get these cost-savers free in this book, you've already saved the cost of several hundred books.

We do a lot of marketing that does work. I know it works because the annual growth in the bottom line tells me it does. We market to:

1. Current patients
2. Emergency patients
3. Newcomers and oldcomers

The previous parts of this chapter tell why. But there is one more element. We try to create a marketing mix that:

1. Keeps us visible
2. Promotes traffic generators
3. Creates a good feeling about us in the community

The last point bears amplification. We have a reputation for promptly seeing anyone in need. We have a reputation for tough competition on price—not cheap; nothing is cheap, just competitive. If anyone has a dental need, we will be easy to find. All of this creates our community sense in our town. It preprograms our patients before we have had a chance to program them in-office.

I've chastised ADA ad campaigns as being so much drivel, which I believe they are. They are being done by a committee—the same committee, I venture, that invented the aardvark. If you read results of studies like the San Diego boondoggle, you will know that any results were created by the ad men, not by patients entering dentists' offices. The whole ad scheme in dental organizations—to the tune of hundreds of thousands of dollars—is a scam of gigantic proportions. But that's another story.

I've raked the ADA brochure *How to Be a Wise Dental Consumer* over hot coals. It's patently ridiculous and an offense to anyone with more than a third-grade education.

This doesn't mean I am anti-ADA. I happen to support it now as I have for decades. I believe in organized dentistry, just as I believe in an organized United States. That doesn't mean, however, that I cotton to all government inanities either.

One of the best items to come out of the ADA is the patient brochure, *Mouthpiece*. Super! Its a great tool that we mail out to thousands of our patients quarterly. It addresses The Hidden Goldmine referred to earlier. It goes to the patient with this feeling: "Here's something free and useful for you because we care about you." Nice. Really nice. It does exactly what we want it to do.

We have a large Yellow Pages ad that keeps us visible when people with "owies" have fingers doing their walking for them. We pack every item of information we can into that ad, including "Man Spricht Deutsch" (one of us speaks German).

We send complimentary introductory coupons to each newcomer to the city through a "Welcome Home" business. People new to town have no prior ties with dentists. They may need service. We feel if we can get them to try us once—which is the absolute most we could expect—we at least have a chance to serve them our powerful first impression.

We have a dental info line with nine tapes on it of special messages about how to choose a dentist, stained teeth, bad breath, affordable dentures, and the like. Consumer health information is not only popular, it is also an obligation of our profession.

Several times weekly, in the City Briefs section of our local paper, we announce quick denture repairs and prompt emergency service.

In the fall of 1983, we took over the city's time and temperature number. A five-second pitch preludes giving; "Dental East (the name of our group) time is ____; the temperature is ____." There are four messages, given in rotation, changed monthly. They will be something like: "Floss daily to detour dental decay and have healthy gums," or "Emergency service is as close as your phone 24-hours daily at Dental East." The first five months we had 1.5 million calls on time and temperature. At five seconds of advertising per call, that's over 2,000 hours of ads.

These are fairly magnificent marketing efforts, but guess what? Our new patient flow stems more from satisfied patients and family-member referrals than from our marketing. And that's the way it's got to be.

What's a new patient worth? We figure our Yellow Pages new patients cost us about $7 each. Too much? No way. A new patient generates something like $60 to $70 of new business. He has family and friends. That's just the dollars and cents.

If he never tries us, he will never learn how great we think we can be for him. Seven dollars for a new patient is one of the best investments that I know how to make. Your stockbroker should give you advice one hundredth as good.

All of our marketing only gives us a one-time shot. If we win with a powerful first impression and follow it by programming our patients with good service, promptly delivered, at fair fees, then we can enjoy the fruits of our labor with PASSION!

13
PROGRAM THE BEST INVESTMENT IN THE WORLD

The price of success is less than the cost of failure.

"Tell me about your poker club, Ed."

"Well, I take ten dollars with me. When I lose that I go home."

How many times do you think Ed wins? Correct. Never. With his attitude, he guarantees his losses. He has programmed himself for defeat. How many times have you gone to Las Vegas or Atlantic City with that same attitude? "When I lose this hundred bucks I'll quit."

How many times did you win? Never, of course. But that's only a hundred. What about the thousands you will fritter away on investment schemes through your productive years? Chances are, if you have normal greedy genes like most of us, at some time you will invest with as poor an attitude as Ed plays poker.

When the first flush of bucks comes your way from dentistry, you will probably think, "Gee, that's easy. Why don't I play some other game? I can certainly play them as well as I play this dental business."

The problem is that being productive in dentistry does not give you expertise to play real estate, tax shelter, oil lease, franchise, stock market, commodity futures, or any of the many exciting games out there in the real world.

Number One Rule to tell Number One Son is, *"Play your own game, Boy*. It is the only game in town for you because it's the only game you know. It's getting repetitious, but none the less still true: You must know the rules for whatever pursuit captures your fancy. That's the first rule of good programming.

Just because you are successful at carving alloy does not give you expertise to carve profits from pork bellies, Krugerrands, Little Miss Muppet Day Care Centers, or Broadway musicals.

For every dentist who has dumb-lucked into a hot outside shot, there are 10,000 who have tried the same stunt and lost their tokus. Their tears would wash every cavity prep in America, forever. Don't let your tears join theirs.

Every investment is some sort of gamble—some greater, some lesser. Generally, enormous risks carry enormous *profit* potential—and enormous *loss* potential. When we coolly rationalize any investment decision, we tend to lose our cool. We allow visions of sugar plums to dance where hard reality should be.

If one of a thousand investors have struck it big, how easily we forget the nine hundred ninety-nine losers. The fact remains, if we lose at an investment, the loss ratio is *not* one percent or ten percent or even ninety-nine percent. From our pocketbook the loss is one hundred percent.

The road to Hell is paved with sure things. Just ask one question of any "guaranteed" deal: "If it's so good, how come I, who knows woefully few of the business rules of the business world, am being invited to join in?"

Sure things are reserved for the pros, if there are any. Dentists are pros at dental health—no more. It's tough to hear, but far less tough than watching $10,000 after-tax dollars, that you sweated out of several thousand buccal pits, tango off to Buenos Aires.

The ultimate goal of an investment is to produce income just as the ultimate goal of an apple tree is to produce apples. It's strange how often we try to grow oranges and bananas on apple trees.

When faced with a choice between income and capital growth, take income first. With enough income, capital growth is assured and becomes a second priority.

Recently, a dentist came up to me during a break in a lecture and told me his wife had just stepped from the room for a moment. "But I want to tell you before she gets back," he said, "how much she needed to hear the importance of investing in ourselves. I need another chair, but she wants a new dining room suite. Now maybe she will understand that with my new chair I will earn her better furniture, faster, and we'll still have the dental chair to produce even more income."

Being the hit man for this dentist is not all that bad. But I asked him why he hadn't gotten the point across before?

He hadn't because he, like most of us, was reluctant to deprive his lady. It takes a great deal of discipline to do. And it *is* difficult for spouses to understand. To this dentist's wife, his new chair was a luxury, not an investment. Her new furniture was a necessity from her point of view.

She had heard him brag about the $1,000 bridge he'd seated that day. She'd translated the bridge into $1,000 of furniture faster than you can say "sold." In his unbridled enthusiasm to let her know how great he was doing in his struggle against poverty, he'd forgotten to help her understand what's left of the $1,000 when it gets to their bank account.

Of course, we all know what happened to it. It shrank. Sixty percent of it went for overhead. That left $400. Two hundred of that went for taxes. That left $200 to spend on furniture or plain things like bread, gas, and diapers. If he invested $20 of the $200 in his investment program, the furniture represented by the remainder could easily be carried home by a one-armed man on crutches.

This has to be the investment starting point: Creating the right mental attitude to understand how a $1,000 bridge shrank between the mouth and the bank. The rules are the same as for all of programming. Know the rules, take a chance, and go at it with PASSION!

Clearing this hurdle, one faces another, "If we had only bought (insert anything: a hot stock, gold, farmland, anything), then we'd be sitting pretty." This implies that all the good investment opportunities have been taken. That's not true either.

There are just as many great opportunities today as there were five, ten, or twenty years ago. But they all take foresight, not hindsight. Don't grieve over lost opportunities; there are more facing you this moment than you can handle. Some of them are good, some of them not so good.

A third investment policy is to divorce pleasure from business. That is, while you may enjoy manipulating your investments, don't use your investment program as a primary source of pleasure. Your first goal is to produce income, then capital growth.

But so often investments become tools of ego, "Gee I've always wanted to own (insert anything that's costly and may not be a good investment)." Fine. Own it if you can. But don't confuse pleasure with business. If you handle your business well enough, there will be plenty of time *and money* for pleasures.

Finally, don't cop out, "By golly, you won't catch me paying 18% for money!" Your father said the same thing when interest rates went from two percent to three percent. If he hadn't, maybe you wouldn't have to work so hard today! Interest rates are always higher than we wish they were, and they're totally irrelevant.

What is relevant is return on invested capital after costs have been deducted. Interest, like taxes, insurance, maintenance, upkeep, depreciation and management costs, is just another cost of doing business. You may as well say, "I won't pay a yard boy more than 60¢ an hour." You will have very long grass if you say that.

Sears, the retail giant, has published a smart little pamphlet that puts percentages in perspective. Their story goes like this: If you buy an item for $100 and repay it at 1½% monthly interest on the unpaid balance (which is 18% annualized), at the rate of $10 paid each month, you will have paid $8.67 interest charges when you make your final payment. This amounts to an actual 9.52% interest payment on the principal over 10 months of payments.

If you understand that, you may want to use those numbers on reluctant patients who balk at 1½% monthly finance charges. It can be a strong selling tool.

Let's review these investment philosophies:

1. Play your own game, not someone else's.
2. Let your helpmate help by telling her/him the truth about the difference between gross production and actual spendable income. They really do want to know. And I'll bet they love you enough to truly care and be a mature partner in your life, not a child for whom you buy trinkets.
3. Don't grieve over lost opportunities; the world is loaded with new ones.
4. Don't play games with business decisions. You will not be your state's next hamburger king. Get your ego kicks out of being good at what you are trained to do.
5. Don't let inflation scare you. It's the backbone of growth and the path to successfully attaining your goal, even if you pay 18% for money—and $1.30 for gasoline.

If you have set these policies in your attitudes, then you may be ready for some of the most pregnant investment counsel you have ever received. These investment gems have three features:

1. They are in your range of expertise. You are a recognized expert in these areas, not a novice. Therefore, you already qualify for the first rule of programming.
2. They generate an income of spendable dollar bills that you can use to create a lifestyle that comforts you and yours and that creates dollars you can leverage into solid growth situations.
3. You have absolute control over these investments. You are not dependent on others for deals that you barely understand. You are not dependent on distant directors or management types to look out for your interests.

These investments will cream any investment you have ever considered.

Quick Return

What would you consider to be a good return on an investment? Would 50% be considered good? Not too shabby.

A $6,000 investment that returns $3,000 would probably rank well with the most demanding of investors. Right?

If there are about 200 working days per year, you would have to receive fifteen dollars of return on each of those days to total $3,000.

Where is this magical investment? It's in your office. Consider that, if you bought a dental chair, operatory light, and handpiece for $6,000, it would only have to yield $15 income for each of those 200 working days to earn at the 50% rate.

Doctor, what procedure would you do for me as your patient that only costs $15? Probably very few. Chances are I couldn't buy a single routine extraction from you for that amount. With your skill such a procedure would take about three minutes of your chair time. And you could sandwich that between anesthesia or material setting times in other rooms.

Consider, too, that with this investment you could expand your services. With an extra chair available for the other 7 hours and 57 minutes of your working day, you can accept those little emergencies, denture adjustments, pain-relief appointments, and other minor but highly important needs that patients present.

You will find that patients you used to turn away because your chairs were appointed solidly all day, can now be seen. You will be stunned to realize how little it takes to please people in distress. And like Androcles and the Lion, you can garner a heroic image, deep appreciation, and new patients and earn far more than a 50% return on your investment.

It's almost unfair that we should earn that much profit on an effort that enhances our ability to serve.

Dentists who shunt away patients with desperate needs "because they are too busy" will one day learn that patients will find an empty chair somewhere. Dentists who do that aren't too busy. They are merely proving that they are inefficient, lazy, ill-equipped, understaffed, or poorly prepared—choose one or more of the above.

Even worse, dentists who are that busy are the same ones who run in circles trying to find investments that yield a tenth of the value and profit that one more chair could create for them.

Here's another thought. Suppose your production is worth $120 an hour or $2 a minute. Many dentists don't have enough mirrors and explorers on hand.

If they have to wait five minutes for such instruments to come out of the autoclave, it costs them ten dollars in lost production. If that happens ten times a month, it's $1,200 of lost production in a year.

And all for the want of $50 worth of spare mirrors and explorers? Incredible? Incredibly true.

Consider an orthopantomograph. If you take as few as two $25 panoramic radiographs each day for those 200 working days, a $10,000 panelipse X-ray machine will return 100% on your investment in the first year alone! From then on the return on investment is pure profit. This doesn't even count how much better you will practice because you'll have more data on your patient.

And there is another sweetener. Ten percent of the value of new equipment purchased can be taken as an investment tax credit. Even leased equipment can qualify for this credit if structured properly.

Remember, there is a large difference between a tax credit and a tax deduction. A deductible item reduces your taxable income. Since you still pay a percentage of your remaining taxable income in taxes, it has only partial value. In a 50% tax bracket, a dollar of tax deduction is worth 50¢ to you.

A tax credit, on the other hand, is reduced directly from taxes you would have paid. Every tax credit dollar, for example, is worth a full dollar. It is *twice* as valuable as a tax deduction.

People Investments

Most dental offices are understaffed. This creates a lot of "stick" dentistry—stick a patient in the chair, stick a needle in his jaw, and stick a magazine in his hand. It does nothing to create good thoughts in patients' minds.

What better investment than to spend $5 an hour in an extra salary to have an assistant visit with the patient while waiting for anesthesia? She could take his mind off his anxiety, find out interesting things in his life to tell you about, visit with him about his dental needs, help elevate his wants to the level of his needs, give your presentations third-person credibility, and generally earn you at least a 200% return on your investment.

But then that's only 200% on $5. Who wants to fiddle around for a lousy $15 profit per hour? Well, that $15 equals $30,000 per year extra profit. If you can employ three extra assistants and have them earn you 200% that's *$90,000 extra profit*. Do I have your attention yet?

For that matter upgrading the salaries of good employees and removing the marginal ones points in the same direction and produces similar results. Investing in an associate to cover expenses while you study or play is a substantially better investment than virtually anything you will find in outside businesses.

Your associate covers your patient's emergency needs, making sure your patients stay in your office, even when you aren't. He gives you someone to counsel with (unless you know everything, of course). He keeps your staff busy and earning their wages. He produces income to pay the light bill. Just as you provide him a source of income, without investment or risk, so does he return the favor.

And Now for the Big One

Own an office building. You can rent it to a nice, solid business owned by a substantial citizen whom you trust and whom you know will treat it well—yourself.

The advantages of renting it to yourself or your professional corporation have been parlayed by many dentists into as fine a real estate investment as can be found. Lenders look kindly on properties that have grade A tenants with stable businesses, such as you.

The result can often be a highly leveraged investment requiring small or minimal upfront money. This allows you to maximize the growth of your money, thereby allowing it to produce income in the form of the rent your professional corporation pays you for the space.

My father is a realtor. He says there are three rules to follow in buying commercial property. The first rule is location; number two is also location; and so is number three.

Once you have selected a good location with a high traffic count (city engineers have counts available for most commercial locations in any city), be certain good parking is available. Every study of dental practice that I have ever seen shows convenience to be the number one factor that people are seeking. Cost is usually second, followed by concerns about pain-free dentistry.

The benefits of income from the property are real. But there are two more benefits: depreciation and appreciation. Both are to be appreciated. Depreciation allows you to write off or deduct a portion of the cost of the building each year from your taxes. Naturally, interest costs, maintenance, taxes, and insurance premiums are all deductible costs, as well.

Appreciation is a gift that property owners receive for growth in property values. When your $100,000 building is finally paid for in 20 years, it may well be worth over $200,000 if appreciation has been adding as little as 5% annually to its value.

When it became apparent in 1979 that we had outgrown our 1,100 square feet of rented office space, I searched for room to expand. An office building was found on an excellent commercial corner across from a twenty-store shopping center. The property had over 3,500 square feet of ground floor space, plus a basement and a second floor with 1,400 square feet of space in each.

A traffic count showed that 38,500 cars passed its front door daily. The parking lot held thirteen cars, with three on-street spaces to the side, and an overflow parking lot next door for 12 more cars. Remodeling costs were fairly reasonable, consisting mostly of modest changes to adapt to our needs. Hookups for suction, nitrous oxide and oxygen, electrical, and plumbing connections were other costs to be borne.

After learning from my attorney that there were no legal problems with the building, such as building code restrictions and past liens, mortgages, or easements, I sought out my accountant.

He investigated the cost history of the building to estimate our costs for taxes, maintenance, and utilities. I had already gone over the property with a contractor to determine if there were any possible surprises in store due to major structural problems.

With clearance from counsel and contractor, my accountant estimated the financial impact of the purchase. His findings were startling and illustrate perhaps best of all what a viable investment an office building for a personal business can be.

The net result of quadrupling our quarters, tripling our parking, and quintupling our productive capacity—from two operatory chairs and one hygiene chair to eight operatory chairs, an X-ray room and a separate hygiene room—was almost beyond belief.

Mike looked up from his calculator and legal pad covered with numbers and announced, "The good news is that Uncle Sam is going to buy this building for you! Your first year net costs, assuming *no* growth in your business, will be exactly $100 more than you are now spending for rent. If your business grows at all, you will end up not only with a net profit but the building will be yours free. There is no bad news!" It was an offer difficult to resist.

Accountants are prone to be conservative and mine proved no exception. Business growth from the expanded service facility wiped out the $100 projected first year loss *during the first day.*

The key elements to this or any transaction are neither the costs of the property nor the interest paid to finance its purchase. If you do not possess programming rule number one, then employ excellent legal, accounting, and contractural advisors. Then you must be assured the proposed property meets your criteria for location, parking, convenience, and convertibility to your needs.

The second consideration is to assess the financial impact of acquiring tax deductions for various aspects of the move, tax credits for other parts of the program, and weighing cash-flow considerations to determine if the project is feasible.

With sound advice from experts who can give you good counsel, these seemingly formidable concerns can be given careful considerations. See how it works?

Know the rules. Those rules you don't know, you hire experts to solve. Take a risk—calculated as all risks must be, but still a risk. And then execute the plan with PASSION!

Surely the world holds exciting investment opportunities. *But the best investment in the world is you.*

14 PROGRAM AFFORDABLE DENTURES

To a man with a hammer, everything is a nail.

—Anon.

The penalty for growing old in America is to become a dental cripple.

Half our elderly try to keep milktoast on the table with an annual income of $3,000 or less. Another 20% live at the mercy of either the state or tolerant relatives. Few have dental insurance. All helplessly watch their dollars shrink to nickels as business and government apply crushing inflationary pressures to their savings.

Many of our elderly have no choice but to consider dental service a luxury. They become either dental cripples, who suffer pain and discomfort, or nutritional cripples, unable to chew because of an unworkable dentition.

The current harvest of elderly did not profit from fluoridation in their lifetime. Dental insurance was unknown during their productive years. In their day dental philosophy encouraged extraction rather than preservation. Today's elderly were victimized and now pay dearly and daily.

The simple truth is *people become edentulous because dentists extract teeth*. Maybe the dentist attempted to counsel preventive attitudes in the patient and maybe he did not. Maybe he was thinking of a quick extraction or denture fee and maybe he was not. But the fact is he either failed to counsel retention of natural dentition or failed to sell its importance. What he did do was extract.

Because of this extraction attitude by dentists in decades past, the elderly have an inordinate prosthetic need today. And because of the financial vice that now grips their lifestyle, they are forced to hobble through their oatmeal on dentures that are often ill-fitting, patched and pasted together with drugstore treatment. Or worse still, they must "gum" it with stiffened ridge tissues that know no denture.

A need this large clamors for solution, if not by dentists, then by others. Until recently the profession has ignored this situation. This has invited aggressive types who, sensing an opportunity of gigantic proportion, have rushed to fill the dental service void.

First, the marketers of proprietary crutches, such as home denture liner kits and denture adhesives, sought to make capital of the situation. The relief they offer is temporizing at best. Often as not their products compound problems by masking tissue destruction and by contributing to bone loss.

Second, others who march under the banner of denturism sought to profit from this dentist neglect. They devised techniques to permit mass delivery of prosthetic appliances at economy prices. They developed marketing strategies that stirred a demand from the edentulous indigent.

Third, denturists have opted to stop serving the public from the back door. They now push for legislation that would dignify their efforts from the front door. Their success in Oregon and Arizona heralds a new age for dentistry. It may be an age we dislike, but it is not an age we can deny.

Brothers and sisters in dentistry: What are we going to do about it?

Crying a lot, in public or private, simply ain't gonna help. You need to understand the nature of the opposition. Denturists make a credible case and wield more influence than you believe.

Often they make dentures that are as good as yours and mine. As a matter of fact, they're sometimes a lot better.

Hard to believe? Believe it. I've visited their operations. I've seen quality prostheses placed by nondentists that would shame many I see that were placed by dentists. They know how to do their job very well. Denturists can get thousands of satisfied customers to testify to that fact, for as many hours as you care to listen.

These are not rinky-dink operations. They function in offices that would put many of our dental offices to shame.

Underestimating one's opposition is the first step to defeat. Do not underestimate the quality of the denturist's product, his empathy with satisfied customers, or his ability to turn public opinion into strong voices to be heard from voting booths.

Consider how the edentulous indigent will believe what the denturists tell him. The message is, "Eyeglasses can be dispensed by optometrists; therefore, dentures can be dispensed by denturists. If an optometrist detects an eye disease, he refers you to an ophthalmologist. If a denturist detects an oral disease, he will refer you to a dentist."

Since 90 percent of the eyeglasses in America are dispensed by optometrists, not ophthalmologists, the denturist makes a compelling case. People readily believe him, as witnessed by his success at the ballot box.

Understand, too, that the profits he makes on quantities of discount dentures are far beyond anything he ever earned working for you. Then there are the ego rewards. He knows that when you seat the handsome dentures he made for you as your lab technician, you will claim all the credit. But if something goes wrong, like the bite or cosmetics, you will blame him.

As your laboratory technician he had to please both you and the patient. And he had little control over whether you took a good impression, marked proper peripheries, registered accurate high and low lip lines, chose a good shade and mold, obtained a satisfactory vertical and jaw relationship registration, and prepared the patient to have a proper mental set to wear dentures.

With you out of the picture, he has control over all those parts of denture construction, and besides that, he gets credit when the patient gushes praise for his new teeth.

The potential denturist faces the prospect of a generous hike in income, a vast increase in community prestige, and the ego justifications of hearing praise for his efforts. The relatively simple task he knows he will have getting his message across to cost-conscious edentulous consumers, the changing business ethics climate of dentistry, and the enormous push for consumerism across the nation each adds impetus to propel him to his goal.

Add up the quality of these carrots that dangle before his eyes, and you know that denturism will not go away.

The story is David and Goliath, Washington crossing the Delaware, and Horatio Alger rolled into one. In the public's eye, the denturist is a white knight out to dismount the "already too-rich dentist monopoly."

Add to these circumstances the fact that the denturist knows more about what you are doing to stop him than you do. He knows that the Council on Prosthetic Services of the ADA has put together a Compilation of Reduced-Fee Denture Techniques to help you learn how to compete with him. He also knows he will cream you, one on one, with any of those techniques, good as they may be.

He knows how badly he beat you in past referendums, despite dentist efforts that cost millions of dollars. He knows the mentality of state legislators who know that they receive little support, if any, from apathetic dentist constituents.

The denturist knows, too, that despite the size and power of the ADA he will take you, one state at a time. He has proven he can. He knows that many dentists don't want to get involved, that many dentists don't care who provides dentures to anyone, that many dentists won't support the ADA, that many dentists are glad anyone besides them can provide denture service to people in lower socio-economic stratas, and that most dentists are so busy planning their next trip to Europe and buying their new Mercedes that they simply don't care about the denture crisis in America. Hard words? Try to think about it objectively.

The denturist is willing and able to spend big bucks to achieve his purpose, but he has found that he really doesn't have to. He has discovered that, if the public is for you, no one can win against you. He will go to jail to win. And he knows how inefficiently most dentists produce dentures, which means they can't compete on his terms.

Finally, he knows that most dentists look on the affordable or reduced-fee denture as a cheapie. He knows that it is the dentist, not the denturist, who has created a market for cheap teeth from South America. He knows that his low-cost dentures probably house better materials than many dentists' custom dentures.

The denturist knows he has a good thing going. His goal is within reach. If you think he will go away or if you think organized dentistry despite its prominence in public opinion polls will carry the day, then you haven't given it much thought.

The only way we can beat a denturist is to beat him at his own game. We want him to play ours, but he won't because he knows the public—now educated to a new credential—will not stand for it. If we are to win, we must play his game. It's the only game in town.

We can beat him at his own game when we become as efficient as he already is, when we learn the time-saving techniques he already knows, when we price our products at a competitive level, and when we impart to our patients that we offer an oral health expertise that the denturist does not possess.

We are, after all, already established in every community in the nation. Our patients already look to us for oral health advice. We have community respect and position. And we have the intelligence to counter at the level that the consumer cares about—the pocketbook.

Dentists have a denture delivery system already in operation that could thwart the push for nondentists to slice off a portion of our services. It could happen if we become efficient and knowledgeable and cut the profiteering out of dentistry. Until we do that, denturists will laugh all the way from the voting booth to the bank. And dentists will cry a lot.

Affordable dentures are not a myth. Affordable denture operations can function within a private general practice. In other words, you don't have to relinquish cost-conscious patients. You can treat them—profitably. Indeed, I have encountered many dentists throughout the country with the fortitude to try to stave off the denturist onslaught. They report some encouraging findings.

First, many people attracted by the economics of affordable denture fees trade up to more profitable (for the dentist) custom dentures.

Second, single-arch denture patients often have an opposing arch with restorative need. An immediate opportunity is there for you to counsel retention of those natural opposing teeth and, of course, to perform salvage procedures.

Third, satisfied denture patients will refer family and friends. Perhaps these patients, who are often into golden years, have more time to visit about their teeth. They often have more family around them to counsel. Or perhaps it is because they accept their edentulous state as a *fait accompli* and are more open to discuss their denture tribulations with others. Whatever the reasons, satisfied denture patients can be excellent referral sources.

Fourth, economical denture operations, properly managed, can be a source of the fair profit needed for any business, including dentistry, to survive.

In 1980 Dental East had grown large enough to afford our own technicians. Before we did so, I traveled from Texas to Michigan, from Ohio to California to watch dentists with successful lab operations as well as denturists, who openly serve the public. It was my first step in programming—to *know the rules.*

From these visits a plan was developed. Mush bites seemed just too chancy, and lack of tryin seemed ludicrous. So, even though these procedures were seen on visitations, they did not seem consistent with the caliber of service we wished to offer.

A technician was hired, equipment installed, and procedures developed to produce, in 24 hours if needed, a consistently high-quality denture. Top of the line materials and teeth were used, and the dentures were flasked. A pin-tracer and tryin became *de rigueur.*

The program worked. We learned the rules. We took a multithousand dollar chance on equipment, salary, supplies, and promotion. And we executed the program with PASSION!

In the trend toward groups as opposed to solo practices, more dental offices will have in-house laboratories. These labs offer more convenience in the form of faster repair, reline, and rebase operations. Convenience in this delivery is as marketable as in any other service we dentists offer.

An in-house laboratory offers an enhanced opportunity to work more closely with technicians, in person, rather than on the phone. It is marvelous to see the change in appreciation and improved technical performance when technicians can, from time to time, be brought to see the patient. Flesh impacts more strongly than plaster.

This bore true in 1982 when we expanded into porcelain with crown and bridge technicians. The doctors gained in appreciation of laboratory services just as the technician gained by observing preparations, working with staff to achieve the best possible impressions, and working with doctors to create a more exact replication of nature's nuances of color.

When a manufacturer develops his own supply lines of raw product to input his operations, the mechanism is called *vertical integration*. Vertical integration in dentistry, by dentists owning and controlling their own laboratory operations, can surely enhance profits.

More importantly, it enhances convenience and quality to the direct benefit of our patients. There is no better reason to pursue these avenues with PASSION!

15 PROGRAM PRESCRIPTION PROFITS

Murphy's Law: *If anything can go wrong, it will.*
O'Tool's Commentary on Murphy's Law: *Murphy was an optimist.*

"Doctor, there's a man here who wants to audit how you dispense drugs. He's from the State. Here's his ID." I paled.

That kind of news can collapse bowels, exhaust breath, and fog vision. Government investigators of any stripe *always* find wrong-doing, widely publicize their policing, extract merciless penances, and always—win. Everyone knows that, don't they?

At Dental East, we dispense drugs—lots of them to lots of people for lots of good reasons. There are also lots of government rules to follow to do it properly. I just knew we had to be missing the boat on several scores, but I didn't know where or how badly we had goofed. Visions of again being a shoe salesman dashed through my mind.

"Bring him right back; I'll be glad to see him." I responded charily. Within, my guts were as knotted as a string of last year's Christmas tree lights. The only thing I could think of that I knew we were doing right was our tight drug security.

That day, and the frenetic days that followed, have passed. We still dispense drugs. Only now we do it according to Hoyle, more particularly, "Uncle Sam" Hoyle. The government man fortunately was rooted in practicality and wasn't a headline-grabber. He straightened us out as neatly as my orthodontist friends adapt an arch wire.

The point of all this is to present for your discovery the goodness that occurs to a dental practice when it cares enough to dispense the very best—correctly. If you do, you need never anguish through moments like those that tore me apart.

Why Dispense?

What factor, more than any other, distinguishes the runners from the also-rans? Asked another way: What is the one factor people choose over all others in reciting why they go to a particular practitioner of these oral arts we call dentistry?

Is it professional skill? Is it charming chairside manners? Is it the size of your advertisements? No, it is none of the above. It is convenience.

Convenience can mean different strokes for different folks. It could be broad office hours, free parking, plentiful staff, colonial reception areas, nifty location, E-Z payment plans, or full service. Full service could mean not referring out every modestly different dental need. It could mean having the latest techniques for deployment. It could also mean dispensing drugs.

Probably, it is a mix of these. We dispense drugs because it is a convenient thing to do for our patients. They are saved the inconvenience of having to go to their pharmacist for antibiotics, pain-relievers, steroids, and nutritional supplements, just to name a few.

By saving them this inconvenience, we also save them time—a highly important commodity. We ensure that the drug is placed instantly in their hands to launch a regimen we feel is important. We save them travel costs, and we price the drugs competitively. These are supremely important pluses.

Studies have shown that many prescriptions are never filled. If we feel strongly enough about a drug need to write a scrip, we want it used—and now. By putting the drug in the patient's hands, we can sooner achieve the benefits we're expecting.

These are sound patient benefits to spring from office dispensing. Since we cannot afford to be a charity, we expect our drug-dispensing to yield a profit. We expect all of the services we deliver to produce a profit. That's a basic part of why we're here.

For the investment the profits are not unsubstantial. Our current inventory of roughly $500 of wholesale-priced drugs turns over about six times annually. At our markups, which compete tightly with the area drug-chain prices, we generate about $2,500 profit after deducting the costs of labeling, packaging, handling, credit, and the drugs themselves.

I know people who would "kill" for a 500% profit on anything. Yet, they fail to offer dispensing as a viable addendum both to patient welfare and to practice welfare. For the most part they grub around with less than two-digit returns on money-market funds. Or they race after leaky tax shelters, dreaming about a nest egg, while a Golden Goose is parked in their own backyard.

How To?

Decide which drugs offer a useful addendum to your practice armamentarium. We chose Motrin 400, Darvon Cpd. 65, Tylenol #3, Tetracycline 500, Penicillin V 500, and Decadron .75. These we package: 6 and 12 of the pain-relievers, 6 of Decadron, and 28, 21, and 12 of the antibiotics.

The 6 and 12 packages of pain-relievers are obviously for shorter or longer potential pain-relief needs. The 6 Decadron packages are for post-surgical swelling reduction and to retard healing when we wish to diminish scar formation, as in lip surgery.

Antibiotics in packages of 21 provide one week of medication at TID. The 28-tablet package provides one week at QID. The package of 12 is for preop: 4 of 500's = 2 GM. stat and then

1 tablet QID for 2 days. Shorter term regimens are packaged as needed. Nutritional supplements are offered in one-month supply bottles.

Once chosen, we ordered initial supplies from wholesale vendors (see the usual mail-order dental suppliers). We provided documentation to them of our various drug licenses (federal and state controlled substances registrations). Then we ordered moistureproof, child-resistant, plastic dispensing bottles from a local medical supply house and had labels preprinted.

Upon receiving our drugs, we fill out a drug log that lists date, drug, amount, expiration date, and lot number. As we fill dispensing packages, we label with the proper data: date, expiration date of drug, lot number, name and strength of drug, directions for use, and our clinic name, address, and telephone number, along with the doctor's name and patient's name.

As we dispense, we fill out a dispensing log that lists: date, name of patient and address (or patient computer number), drug, and amount. Each day a staff doctor signs the dispensing log. On May 31 in odd-numbered years, we are required to do an inventory count of remaining drugs.

That's simple enough. Far less complicated than finding a fast-food franchise that is a good investment. And, however complicated it may seem at the outset, it is merely a matter of taking one step at a time. Once done, it only requires normal, daily vigilence and prudence. No big deal, for all the patient and practice benefits it returns.

The "State" Man

I won't bore you, or embarass myself, with how many ways we violated these staple paradigms. But we were fortunate enough to have an investigator who knew we consciously wanted to comply, but were doing so with an ineptitude matched only by *Peanuts'* Charlie Brown or *Bloom County's* Opus.

He helped us square ourselves with the federal and state world. Not only did he help, but he showed us case by case where these laws protect not only our patients but us as well.

For example, a moistureproof container prevents packaged drugs from absorbing moisture from the air, which reduces their useful shelf life. Penicillin in tablet form in a moistureproof container has a shelf life in months. In solution, however, it breaks down in a matter of hours. Moisture-riddled penicillin will not have the same efficacy as the more stable dry form. That's only one of many thoughts he shared with us.

He also showed us how dispensing logs may be of inestimable value in the unlikely event a particular lot number of a drug is recalled by the manufacturer. This is an important safeguard for our patient's welfare as well as our own.

He introduced us to stickon labels for dispensing bottles that included: *"DO NOT DRINK ALCOHOLIC BEVERAGES when taking this medication"* for penicillin, since alcohol ties up the drug and dilutes its efficacy; *"May cause Drowsiness or Dizziness"* for Motrin, Darvon Cpd .65, and Tylenol #3, for obvious reasons; *"Do not take Dairy products, antacids, or iron preparation within one hour of this medication"* for tetracycline, since the calcium with milk and dairy products binds them up.

Because we didn't have an active dispensing log, thousands of charts had to be examined to record each of the past two years' dispensations—a not inconsiderable expense in terms of staff labor. But never again.

If you begin to offer drug-dispensing to your patients and if you follow these simple rules, then when your receptionist announces that a man is here to audit your drug accounts, you will welcome his presence. You won't care if you are as lucky as I was to have a rare, real human being wielding the government's pencil. And in the interim, both you and your patients will enjoy benefits of thoughtful practice functions that offer a new level of convenience.

16 PROGRAM BUCKS IN YOUR BANK ACCOUNT

The Golden Rule of Arts and Sciences: *Whoever has the gold makes the rules.*

A lot of dentists think they have sold, let's say, a three-unit bridge when the patient says, "Yes, let's do it." Some dentists think they have sold the bridge when it is seated. But smart dentists know the truth. The bridge isn't sold until the bucks are in your bank account. A sale isn't complete until it's paid for, and that is number one rule for all seasons.

You've heard it and read it, and I have too, that if we will but go on a cash basis, our worries will end. One hundred percent collections is truly an awesome thought. But it is a short-circuited thought. That's because it presumes your growth rate will go on endlessly. And I Doubt that with a capital "D."

No business ever achieved its majority without the proper use of credit. That's "use," *not* "abuse." What we're going to discuss now is how to avoid collection heartache and how to program collections. The concept is so simple, I don't understand why so few do it.

Collection problems are the dentist's fault, not the patient's fault. Oh, hey, that's heavy metal. To chastise Dr. Nice Guy for a patient's failure to fulfill his half of the contract seems unfair. But it's true.

Until you accept that simple fact, you will anguish in vain over collections. Because collection problems begin before you ever touch a tooth.

If you have explained your credit policies at the outset, within five minutes of when a new patient crosses your threshold; *if* you have checked the credit reliability of your patient; and *if* you have set a payment program you both can live with, you will collect 96% of all production.

Why not 100%? Because 4% is the cost of doing business. Four percent is your donation to community (professional) responsibility to serve all mankind—even the destitute. It's fair, if controlled and kept at no greater than 4%.

If perchance you were collecting 100%, I'd guesstimate you are missing at least half the new business that should come your way. Ninety-six percent of $400,000 gross business is still more than 100% of $200,000—don't let anyone tell you otherwise.

But I suppose we are dentists because we are professional nitpickers. And people who pick nits for a living usually get hung up on that $16,000 (4%) loss of $400,000. Those who do never achieve it.

This does not mean we allow our patients to walk all over us. We don't . We set our policies and do everything we can to entice people who fit those policies to visit us.

One of those policies is that you are a dentist, not a banker. If a patient wants credit dentistry, you give him credit *options*, none of which includes *your* pocketbook. That's tough, to be sure, but it's the *only* sane way to stay sane and solvent.

Here's how we do it. The method and the numbers were the same a few short years ago when we were smaller.

Again, this may not be the *correct* way or the *best* way, and it surely isn't the *only* way; but it *works* for us. Here's how we program patients to cooperate with our plans to pay our bills on time.

Our credit policies are announced when a patient calls for service, "The first visit is expected to be paid for at the visit. Other credit arrangements may be made for later visits." This is the initial program phase. It may weed out a few who didn't intend to pay. If so, so much the better.

Our credit policies are put in the patient's hands when he signs in, fills out our health questionnaire, and receives our patient brochure. In addition, our discount policies are explained on the health *and* finance questionnaire, which we place in his hands. Signs in our office state:

1. Payment Is Expected the Date Services Are Rendered
2. 5% Discount on Services When Paid the Date of Service

These signs are placed strategically so patients cannot miss them.

At the chair, costs are estimated by our dental assistants. The doctors rarely ever do so. We'll come back to that point later. After we have collected the data we need to determine treatment options, I lay it on the patient at once. Afterward, the chairside DA takes over, completes the explanations in lay language, and fills in the costs. This gives the patient a few minutes, between being told the costs and going back to the receptionist to make appointing and financial arrangements, to think about it.

Now the patient has the information he needs to make a treatment decision based upon his ability to pay. He runs the show. It's his mouth, his future, and he has the right to direct that future with good or faulty (perhaps in our view) decisions.

My role is to learn his problems, suggest solutions, and then to do what he wants. His role is to decide intelligently what he wants, in terms of what he can afford, and then to pay for what he chooses.

Once he has decided what he wants, he chooses a plan that both works for him and creates office income for us. We give him numerous payment options.

First, there is the 30-day account. People can use this who show that they have not abused it elsewhere (credit check) or have established a satisfactory payment history with us.

Second, there are the Mastercard, American Express, and Visa accounts: "Want to pay only five percent of your balance per month? Use MC or Visa." If their credit line on those cards is used up, we go for a "zero" card, which is an additional credit line that MC or Visa may issue in this circumstance. If MC or Visa refuses them, who am I to presume that I know more about credit than these professionals?

Third, there are bank plans—a dental bank plan at one bank in town and a conditional sales contract that we have established with another. We never cosign with the patient.

Fourth, if a patient says, "I want to make payments to you, Doc." I say, "Great! Do it. And when you have paid us $50 or $100, I'll then do $50 or $100 worth of work for you." But the patients pay us *before* I go out on a limb for them. It is exactly what they have asked for—a time payment program. It meets my requirement to get paid, too. The only difference (and it's a biggie) is that they *pay me before I do the work*—not after.

With credit programs like these, it is difficult to get in trouble on collections. But there are still several possibilities: the emergency patient without funds ("left my checkbook at home"), the "I'll get paid Friday" patient, and the insured patient.

For insured patients we accept an insurance guarantee as payment in full and use all of our credit policies (above) on the patient's share. We fill out the insurance form and submit it. We do not let the patient do this because patients are not as interested in my financial health as I am. These are submitted within 24 hours of when the work is completed. Our computer kicks them out in one or two seconds.

If patients say they want to wait and see how much the insurance will pay, we give them two options: (1) They may pay the entire amount, and we will forward the insurance check to them; or (2) we will fill out an insurance guarantee form and let the insurer tell us what they will pay before the work is done.

Our statement to them goes like this, "The only way we can accept the insured portion as payment in full is to accept estimated patient-portion payment at the outset."

Did you pick up on the most revolutionary thought in dental insurance since dental insurance began? Did you catch the word "guarantee"? It may do for you the great things it has done for us.

I don't know who dreamed up *preauthorization,* but if he was a dentist, he shouldn't claim any credit for it. My guess is it was an insurance type. That word was banned in my office long ago. It should be banned from Webster's dictionary and every dental office in the land.

We *never* say to a patient, "When the insurer (or state welfare) gives us preauthorization, we'll go ahead with this work." That statement plays directly into the insurer's hand and hurts you more than you know.

Preauthorization implies that the insurer has a say in your patient's treatment, which it does not, and that the insurer is the patient's benefactor, which it is not. Your patient *earns* his dental insurance. He negotiated for it, and he pays a share (deducted from his paycheck) for it. The insurer is simply a bank from which the insured draws the benefits he has earned and to which he is entitled.

That's why we banned preauthorization from our vocabulary. We use the term *guarantee,* which brings it all into a perspective that puts you in your proper role. Here's how.

"Sally, when we have the insurance *guarantee,* we will proceed with the work. Then you will know exactly what they will *guarantee* to pay and exactly what your share will be." Sometimes, when I am positive that a guaranttee will be forthcoming, I go ahead at once.

For the emergency patients who have no money, the rules are modified. We see them, of course. It would be difficult to sleep with oneself if we denied our skills to the destitute. I cannot imagine how any dentist could be so heartless.

We try to collect from the announced destitute, but not for long. We give it a shot at the reception desk and then give it another shot with a statement. And when that fails, I send this letter:

```
Dear ________,

  My bookkeeper tells me that you have not paid
your $_____ balance due for our services. I'm
surprised, but there must be a reason. Is it one
of the following?

  _________  I am unemployed/on strike.

  _________  I am dissatisfied with your ser-
             vice because ____________________
             _________________________________.

  _________  I intend to honor this debt. I do
             not want it on my credit history.

  If you feel we were unfair in our fees, please
reduce them to whatever you think is fair, pay
that amount, and we will consider it paid in
full. We want to be fair. At the same time we
have costs that must be met, too.
  We value you as a very important person, our
patient. We do not want this debt to hurt our
friendship.

Sincerely,
```

Collection agencies and small claims courts are a no-win situation. They are proof that we have failed to do a complete job for our patients in helping them to fulfill their obligation to us.

Chairside Presentations

A few pages ago it slipped out that we do chairside presentations. That statement is 99% true. Only rarely do we schedule private office presentations. And then it's usually when we either need further study or more data from outside sources (specialist consultations, consultations with other staff doctors, credit information, and the like). Most presentations are done chairside, and our staff plays a large role in them.

Since our explanations of most procedures are brief—22 seconds for a space maintainer and 50 seconds for a root canal filling—and couched in lay language, chairside assistants can handily discuss areas they feel fairly sure the doctor will want discussed. They can begin programming a patient for the sale. Often, after the doctor has seen a patient and collected records (such as health questionnaire, B/P recording, drug regimens, X-rays, exam findings), a smart chairside assistant can complete the entire sale.

The doctor then assures that his diagnosis and treatment plan are proper, that no unanswered questions remain, and that the patient fully understands the proposed treatments, the costs, and has been given an opportunity to begin thinking about how he is going to pay for it.

To be sure, many practice management experts advise otherwise. It has been fairly traditional to counsel the doctor to set aside a special time to do so. In my view, that is a complete waste of a doctor's productive time.

In many ways it follows the old principle of "never do too much dentistry at one appointment" and "never do it too quickly." People who counsel those practices are trying to build confidence in the *doctor,* not the patient. We start with the knowledge that we will advise to the best of our abilities and that what we suggest will be fairly priced.

Further, we develop treatment plans in concert with the patient for they are the ones who pay the freight. It's their money they spend; it's their future; it's their responsibility. We have to know what they want, what they are willing to invest in themselves, and their attitudes. To find out these things requires questions. From answers to our questions we develop a profile of the patient that helps us serve them more intelligently. It helps us suggest treatment plans that fit with their wishes.

Of course, if patient wants are inconsistent with needs we say so—point blank, on the spot. But we lay it on them immediately, without clever waltzing. We are not into playing games with things as precious as dental health.

That's exactly how we deliver services in an orchestrated harmony of action, four to six skilled hands tending every patient service.

We use head and hand signals for most operations. We do not want a negative word to intrude on the pleasant experience our staff is dedicated to delivering.

In the past, we have used a stopwatch to time our procedures so we can more accurately estimate appointment scheduling and better manage our time.

Each element of patient services is part of our total programming efforts to create happy patients who feel real enthusiasm for the value of our service.

PASSION! makes it happen.

17 PROGRAM YOUR TIME

Segal's Law: *A man with one watch knows what time it is. A man with two watches is never sure.*

Few gnawing feelings are worse than having too much month left at the end of your money—and then having a two-hour bridge prep disappoint. Let's discuss cancellations (CA's), broken appointments (BA's), and nighttime emergency callers. Each has a unique hold on the use of our time. Each will tolerate a certain measure of programming.

It probably sounds strange to say, but some CA's are probably good for us. That flies in the face of the Puritan work ethic, which says we have to be drudges every waking moment, but I'll say it anyway: *There is some good that can happen during unplanned downtime!*

Writing and lecuring are pleasant avocations for me. Downtime lets me pursue plans for both these interests. But since I concentrate them on our profession, there are double benefits.

Writing out my thoughts helps me codify my thinking and clarify my intent. Doing so has helped our office in goal-seeking. I show these writings to my staff and my associates, who then better understand my direction. I share them with my colleagues, just as others have shared with me in the past.

Downtime gives us a chance to ask ourselves questions. When did you last sit in your reception room as your new patient does and really see it? Do you offer hot chocolate, coffee, and tea? Do you have female-oriented magazines? Is there abundant greenery? Does the scene seem peaceful and orderly, yet warm and nonthreatening?

During downtime we can assess our patient brochure, check our credit policies, go over office policies, and update training manuals. Our staff can catch up on those many tiny details that we want to be perfect, to set us apart from the herd.

Downtime keeps us humble, too. Maybe that is the grandest benefit of all.

I'll expand briefly on a couple of these points. Over 80% of all dental appointments are made by women, therefore the female-orientation of our office. People trust professionals more when there are plentiful numbers of green things growing about. A cup of coffee or tea literally breaks the ice in patients' attitudes about us. We use jars of powdered products and a large urn of hot water.

Our credit policies should be clearly exposed, in succinct language, to each new patient within five minutes of their entering our practice in order that we may lay the groundwork for collection efficiency later.

Looking at our office through our patient's eyes is not an exercise to fill time. It's a meaningful method of creating a selling, receptive environment. These seemingly minor points are not minor at all because our patients both choose us and reject us on the strength of trivial emotional biases that we create.

They tell me in Las Vegas that oxygen is pumped into the air conditioning systems so that gamblers will not tire so readily. There are no clocks on gaming room walls, and every sort of luxury is available at your elbow at all times. Why? To increase the odds for the house. That is precisely what we do when we get the "gift" of downtime. We try to use it as time to stack the odds of patient acceptance in our favor.

A few years ago my eldest daughter was a hostess at a fine restaurant. How complicated can that really be? Sounds fairly simple to me. But wait.

Cyndee's job description was twelve pages long, typewritten, and single spaced! Now isn't it at least of equal value to sell abundant living through fulfilled dental health as it is to sell crab legs and prime rib? I agree with you. It is.

But how can it be done effectively without a plan and a goal? Our office policies tell what we want to accomplish and the method we intend to use to achieve that goal. I will wager that not one of the last hundred dentists to go bankrupt had either a plan, a goal, or office policies.

"Oh I'm too small for all that monkey business!" is the response I've heard—too often. It springs from a harbored sentiment in the profession that says, "When I grow, I'll hire more staff, get larger and better offices, and secure some really good (or really needed) equipment." That attitude displays a pitifully myopic view.

It is akin to saying upon opening a practice, "As soon as I get a patient, I'll rent an office, hire staff, and buy my equipment." The time to grow is *before* it happens because, if you wait until *after* it happens, it will *never* happen.

Downtime, well spent, can be an enormous practice plus.

Effective Scheduling

To start with, if you want patients to respect your time, you first must respect theirs. Everything that could possibly have been written about that point has already been pressed in very old ink. But to help us at Dental East perform as we want to do, we use several devices.

When a patient registers in with the receptionist, that fact is announced on the intercom, "Jim Black, 2:30, is here." Now, the ball is in the chairside DA's court. Her task is to get the patient to the chair in ten minutes. Sometimes I inadvertently slow her down by extending a procedure on a prior patient.

When she sees that, she announces to me, "Red alert in chair two." This tells me I'm dragging and better get back on schedule. Or she will use the same phrases if a patient has a 3:30 appointment elsewhere following his 2:30 appointment with us. I then know I have to perform, not talk about it, not excuse myself with all the lame excuses you and I have both been taught, but perform. Get that patient in and out on time, not give him the old stuff about, "I didn't rush my last patient, and I won't rush you."

Another safeguard to avoid downtime is to pack the schedule tightly. I have a simple rule that I teach my receptionists, "Fill tomorrow." Don't show me an appointment book beautifully half-filled for the next six weeks. I get no jollies bragging to colleagues that I'm booked solid two months ahead. I'm not.

Anyone who is booked that far ahead isn't a competitor in the dental marketplace anyway. He is your absolutely least worry. You should hope that every colleague in your town is booked that way because, if they are, you are sitting on a gold mine of opportunity. Fill one day at a time, and all those tomorrows will add up to a golden future.

I help my receptionist when I know she's running into a snag on filling an appointment. It happens. But she *must* communicate that fact to me so I can do something about it. When I am told of near-term appointment vacancies (or near-term cancellations), I then can say: "Ginny (patient), I want to see that tooth as soon as you and I can meet again at the chair. Connie (chairside DA), do you think there might be an opening this afternoon (or tomorrow or whenever)?"

My receptionist soon learns conversation that doesn't make it seem like we live in Desperation City "Ginny, you're in luck. I've just had an opening for this afternoon at two."

Need it be said that no patient ever, ever, ever sees our appointment book? No, I didn't think I had to say that.

The telephone is one tool we employ to help fill sudden gaps. First, we call and remind all of the following day's patients. You can easily justify extra salary expense for this person if she only jogs a couple of memories a day. She will. And she will easily earn her keep, too. Also, she will discover if an appointing error was made—the appointment card said Tuesday and should have said

Wednesday. Or she may discover, "Oh, gee! Aunt Mabel just died, and we're on our way out of town now." Learning this saves you great grief, and it's not over Aunt Mabel's demise.

Second, we use the telephone to follow up on broken appointment patients whose charts are kept handy for that purpose. Also, we regularly call through the BA's to scout for people who want to try again.

Third, a standby list of patients with need can be useful to fill gaps in tomorrow or afternoon cancellations. I've never been a big believer in this one, but my staff uses it more than they let me know they do. So it's working for me probably better than it should, despite my attitude.

Every time a CA or BA occurs, we chart it in bright red ink on the patient's chart. This lets us see patterns develop because people who habitually break or cancel appointments do it, well, habitually.

We never give these people the first appointments in a morning or an afternoon. If we do and they cancel or break, we're stuck. There is little chance to do anything about it. But if they fail later in the day we (1) may receive a little lead time from them before they fracture their appointment or (2) discover their absence a few minutes into their appointed time. We can do something about these events.

The somethings we can do are what I call creative appointing. It took awhile to learn. I'll save you the agony of having to learn it the slow way, like I did.

A recall schedule can be an excellent feeder for empty operative chairs. If I check a recall and know I have a spare chair, I'll say, "Bill, I've got time to do those fillings right now. Shall we save you the time and inconvenience of returning later?" Always mention the *patient benefit* in the same breath.

A prompt emergency policy helps, too. We see every emergency the same day they call if that is their pleasure. Those patients are great for filling holes in schedules. This is one of our most important policies for growth. It's about the last policy I'd drop if I had to drop a policy.

You also might be able to expand work for a prior appointee when an unexpected schedule breakdown occurs.

One final trick I learned from the airlines. Do you know how they handle no-shows and last-minute cancellations? They overbook their flights. We overbook our chairs when the opportunity or need arises.

We will book two habitual BA or CA patients for the same time. If both show, we do half as much for each patient. "Nancy, there's more work on that tooth than I thought. But I'm not going to rush it. I want it right and you do, too. We'll have to make another appointment to finish your work." Not a word is said about BA's or CA's.

There is enough anxiety and self-inflicted torment in dentistry without us laying more on the patient. Of course, for repeat violators my receptionist may call their history to their attention and invite them to "shape up or ship out." Sometimes the best offensive is a strategic retreat. Let those patients muddy up someone else's water.

The one thing I would never do is charge for a broken appointment. That policy perfumes the air and has no place in any office I can think of.

With a refreshed attitude about the value of downtime, with office teamwork to address schedule breakdowns, with a policy that addresses only the near term, with a prompt emergency policy, and most of all, with a creative doctor who actively enters the schedule program, rather than passively accepting what his receptionist dishes out, you will smooth out your schedule, your cash flow, and your nerves.

If you don't know where you are or where you're going, you're already there!

18 PROGRAM PEOPLE WHO GO "OUCH" IN THE MIDDLE OF THE NIGHT

Boren's First Law: *When in doubt, mumble.*

Emergencies self-describe as never occurring at convenient times. When the cares and demands of the day (or week) are tucked to bed, people have time to concentrate on a concentrated problem somewhere within them. Dental problems, occurring close to the brain, can become high priority on weekends, holidays, and evenings.

If the number of general dentists who offer 24-hour answering service is a measure, the common method of treating odd-hour emergencies is to avoid them. Some dentists go to the length of having an unlisted home telephone number! That is probably the ultimate in avoidance. My guess is that patients who learn that about their dentist figure out ways to avoid him just as successfully.

"Doctor, I need to have this tooth pulled right now!" The plea is frantic and certainly seems genuine. The diagnosis may even be correct. But at 2 a.m. it is difficult to deal with.

Try to *never* go to your office after hours. Problems with druggies, muggers, opportunistic women who may cry "rape," and thieves who draw you from your home to strip it while you're gone are simply not smart encounters.

If we have to go to the office, we know the person in need. If there is a fraction of a doubt, we call the local police who willingly meet us there to check out the validity of the call. Preferably, we take someone with us, anyone to obviate some of those potential problems.

Better still, don't go at all. Does that sound heartless? Not at all. It is simply prudent. My rejoinder to patients who call is, "I'd be glad to see you, but I cannot get staff at night. And I cannot serve anyone properly without my trained staff." Dentistry is just too complex today to muck along alone.

This doesn't mean we don't gladly advertise and pursue emergency services with vigor. We do. We display ample notice of 24-hour emergency service availability in our Yellow Pages ad. Here's how we do it. When a person calls, their complaint is usually either pain, trauma, or discomfort (as in dentures).

For pain, I prescribe appropriate medications. If I doubt the patient, I may give him something mild, very few of whatever I prescribe, and then alert the pharmacist to be sure the person can produce a picture ID. He will also check to see if the patient is on a drug alert list, which our pharmacists keep as a ready reference. Another device is to develop, from the patient's answers, the probability of infection and prescribe antibiotics, checking first for allergies with all prescriptions, of course.

Few druggies will buy an antibiotic prescription just to obtain three Tylenol #3's, for example. The economics of street drug trade won't support that program. This becomes an effective safeguard, especially when the pharmacist is alerted to not dispense one drug alone; both prescriptions *must* be purchased. If retail pharmacies are closed at that hour, the hospital pharmacy will dispense at night.

"Have you had swelling or soreness in your jaw?" "Have you had drainage or excess pressure?" Those are questions that lead to infection probabilities. My response is that I do not remove highly infected teeth until the infection subsides "because extraction might force bacteria into your bloodstream and cause another infection in your heart, liver, kidneys, or elsewhere."

Patients suffering a traumatic incident, who need an oral surgeon, are referred for proper service. Those with broken teeth are told that proper treatment requires full staff, not me alone. So we dispense some ideas to help them, medication if needed, and offer kindly encouragement. Many callers only want to talk with someone knowledgeable, and your telephone assurance can often be enough to ease their anxieties and allay their fears. Proper service, even done a day or two later, is better than slapdab service promptly rendered.

Applying a pledget of cotton soaked in oil of cloves, adapting warm paraffin over the exposed tooth area, and avoiding hot and cold food and drink are some of the tips we suggest to help the patient through the anxious moments until we can see them and serve them properly. Patients with denture discomfort are advised to use topicals such as Benzodent®, warm saltwater mouth rinses, or leave the denture out until we can treat it during regular office hours.

Routinely, we tell these off-hours emergency callers to show up at the office the next working day so we can follow up with our treatment. At that time they can be properly introduced into our practice, be told our office policies (for their acceptance or rejection), and be cared for infinitely better than I can do it alone during off times. "When you call the office be sure and tell Susan that you talked to me and that I insisted you been seen right away." That's the phrase that helps them feel they have an inside track to my services.

This approach cuts our off-hours emergency office visits to nearly zero. Yet, we still dispense comfort and hope to patients we want to see. It lets them know we care about them too much to do slipshod service, which I surely would be performing if my staff were not attending the patient with me.

There seems to be some sort of guilt complex prevalent among dentists. It says, "It's my fault my patients have problems." Well, it simply isn't our fault that patients have emergencies or recurring problems. You are the source of relief for your patients' discomfort. But don't confuse your role and accept a burden of guilt for how people goof up their dental health.

Most emergency problems that do occur are the result of patient neglect. That brings us to the final point I would make. We never chastise a patient for neglecting himself. He already knows that. What useful purpose is served by exacerbating that wound?

Dealing with emergencies by prudent programming and not allowing patients to reprogram us to their frailties can make emergency service a plus in dental practice.

It can be done with PASSION!

19
PROGRAM PLEASURE IN PRACTICE

When an optimist wears out his shoes, he just figures that he is back on his feet.

—Anon.

"Jerry! How's it going?" We hugged hands. I hadn't seen Jerry is 26 years, since we graduated from dental college.

"Swell, Schmitty. Only eight more years and I hang it up."

"No kidding? Then what?" I asked.

Jerry waggled his hand. "Who knows? But it sure as hell won't be this lousy job!"

I was stunned. Jerry's comment implied that his whole life wasn't worth a hill of spit. The past 26 years had to have been a chore, the next eight were a write off, and retirement was anything but the profession we pursued. What had soured one of the eager grads we both once had been?

If anything, practice gets more delicious for me every day. My program simply allows no room for any other thought. It was a Saturday seminar when we met. Every weekend, every holiday, every vacation for years has found me eager to get back—not to the salt mine—but to the salt that's mine, my practice.

I've thought about Jerry's attitude a lot since then; if what I see in the professional press is an indication, Jerry has more company than our profession likes to admit. Stress, boredom, executive fatigue, and our calling's dismal lifeline statistics all point to a problem of large proportions.

Perhaps other indicators are "busyness" conferences, practice management seminars all over the place, and high readership of practice management and economics journals. If these gauges are read correctly, I believe they report that a swell of professional discontent exists throughout the land.

I refuse to be stressed. I don't really know what it's all about.

I surely don't get bored. We bring in hundreds of new patients every month and have a staff of thirty to handle them. Gosh! There's so much excitement going on, no way could I get bored. And fatigued? I'm down to three seven-hour days and two five-hour days. Shoot, I can do that on my ear—with lots of time off to travel, speak, and do all sorts of fun things. Stressed? Bored? Fatigued? Where? When? Why?

As for busyness conferences—sorry. Go ahead without me. We're much too busy with patients and things we enjoy to find the time to attend.

My question is why are so many of my colleagues overlooked, underbooked, and marking time until they are boxed? I know why I'm happy, and I think it's the same reason so many are not. I'm fearful most of my colleagues think they will be happy when they get into big bucks. If you've gleaned that from this book then I've misled you.

Big bucks never bought happiness—never ever. What is neat is the crux of the whole matter. It makes getting up and charging into the office a joy. And it's so simple, I wonder why no one else has ever said it before.

I love my patients.

The great truths of life, you'll recall, are always simplistic. Nothing could sound simpler than "love your patients." But just a minute, I said the concept is simple—carrying it out is not necessarily all that simple. It requires a great deal of thought and a vigorous amount of practice. But payday is oh so sweet.

We love our patients so much they beat down our doors to keep us thriving. It could happen to you. And when you truly orient your practice to this concept, you'll never regret it.

Love

It starts with the greatest four-letter word in the world—*love*. Now love is a funny word. It's funny because everybody thinks he's an expert at it, and almost nobody is. It's funny because the same people who readily recognize they have to practice to become a good golfer, fly fisherman, or bowler believe they were born knowing all about love. Now that's really funny.

It's funny, too, because it's the *only* avenue to happiness. There is absolutely none other. If you had all the money you could dream of, tell me how you'd be a better person? What part of your lifestyle would it enrich? You would be happy for maybe three minutes—then what? Then you'd want someone with whom to share those possessions, travel, meals, entertainments, and security. Enter love.

If you think you can buy that love with all your money, dream on. Love isn't, hasn't, and never will be for sale. You'll be the loneliest one-night-stand in town.

Understand, too, one more thing. The opposite of love is not hate—it's apathy. Ask your neglected spouse. Or someone else's if yours isn't. If he/she isn't neglected, yours is the rare marriage. With our national divorce statistics, it isn't hard to draw that conclusion.

I Love My Staff

Try it out on your staff. If you are dropping your full love load at home, your spouse wouldn't dream of jealousy. He/she will be too busy dreaming of how they are going to make you happy next. You won't believe how inventive they will be when they know—truly know—that you are wildly in love with them. And the neat thing is that you can give every ounce of your love away and still have it all left within you. Incredible bargain!

I promised I'd tell you what we do in these regards to show how much we care about the staff. We've already noted how we program our staff to complement our office goals.

Sure we pay competitively well and have the usual fringes, but we try to make it fun. We try to pop surprises on them and make them happy in the knowledge that we love them enough to spend time and effort to bring them a smile or a simple pleasure.

Example: Whenever we shatter an office production record, I find something nice to give my staff. Once it was Calvin Klein jeans for all. I made a deal with a local store—25% off for our group—then told the women to go get their sizes. Once it was sweaters with our office logo stitched on. Once it was office T-shirts. Once it was shoes. Another time, western shirts.

On St. Patrick's day a box of bright green carnation corsages shows up, the same on St. Valentine's day except they are red. During Dental Assistant's Week last year, on Monday I gave them a huge tin of KarmelKorn, on Tuesday donuts for all, on Wednesday candy, on Thursday huge trays of sweet rolls, then on Friday the clincher—scales for the staff lounge!

It was a delicious joke and showed my staff that I truly cared, that I had spent some time and thought on them. I do it for the simple reason that *they make everything possible for me!* I just can't love 'em enough.

I Love My Patients

I once published an article on advertising for health-care professionals. I promptly received a vituperative letter from a doctor in Texas. His thrust was that he believed I didn't care about the dignity of our profession. I didn't know how to answer him until one morning a thought struck and I made a long distance phone call, then wrote him a reply.

In my letter I said something to this effect:

> You say I don't respect the dignity of our profession, Doctor. But I submit there is a greater dignity which I do respect, and that is the dignity of humanity.
>
> If you will call our office and tell my receptionist that you have a severe problem and no money, she will ask, "How soon can you get here?"
>
> This morning, I called your office and told your receptionist I had a severe problem and no money. She told me to get lost.
>
> I submit, Doctor, that a respect for the humanity of man is of far greater import than a self-serving, misplaced, and misguided respect for our profession. I do respect our profession, but my priorities are in order.

Love in our practice is to never put down our patients. In this manner we program more positive responses in our patients. Here's one way—I never wear jewelry at the chair. There's a simple reason for that; I want the patient to know our concern is for his health, not my wealth.

My office desk is an architect's drawing board, shoved against the wall. Its function is to be out of the way, rather than a throne behind which I reign. It allows me to go face to face with my patients on an equal-footing basis.

There are no wall plaques of degrees and similar ilk dressing up my private office. My patients already know I graduated from dental school. They know I've chaired a bunch of committees and paid my community dues. I needn't remind them of such things and run the risk of suggesting self-importance.

For the past three years, we have worn designer jeans and nice tops to work. This includes all my staff, my two associates, and myself. It puts us on a comfortable level with our patients. Never once has a single patient objected to these outfits. On the contrary, on the day we began to wear them, three of my most anxious patients volunteered, "You know, Doc, I feel more relaxed and comfortable today. I think it's what you guys are wearing!" Need there be a better reason?

When we sell, we use patient language with words any ten-year-old can understand. My patients are aware that we know the five-dollar words. I don't need to get my jollies by impressing them with the foreign language of science when simple and common words work just fine. Here are a few ways we talk patient language rather than doctor lingo.

When we sell a space maintainer, the talk goes like this:

> Betty, Jimmy's baby tooth has been lost too soon. That molar should have lasted until Jimmy was in fifth grade and saved a space for a new tooth. Now that it has been removed, Jimmy's jaw will shrink unless we put in a little brace to save the space. [22 "selling" seconds long.]

And when we sell a root canal filling, the talk goes like this:

> Bill, you have a dead nerve in that tooth. Your body will treat it just like it would treat a splinter left in your finger—it will fester. To prevent that, we have to take the dead nerve out. We can do that two ways. We can pull the tooth, which for sure gets rid of the nerve, but that's sort of like throwing the baby out with the bath water. There's another way we can do it. We can just take the dead nerve out and leave the tooth. We do that like you would take the wick out of a candle from one end. That leaves a hollow tube, which we fill. And that's what a root canal filling is all about. [50 "selling" seconds long.]

Before an extraction I grasp the patient's shoulder and say:

> Frances, you have two nerves going to this tooth. One tells you about pressure, which is the same nerve that tells you my hand is on your shoulder. The other tells you about pain. I can put the pain nerve to sleep—you won't feel any pain—but I cannot put the pressure nerve to sleep. So you will feel pressure and movement and hear a slight crunchy sound.

And then, if needed, I add:

> I believe this tooth will come out in pieces, but no problem—we know how to do that. [20 seconds.]

When our thoughts are simply stated, few will misunderstand them. They reinforce our patients with full information and do not put a patient down by using words that intimidate. My staff, too, can give these explanations in confidence, freeing doctor's time for more productive efforts.

My patients enjoy hearing my staff give them information far more than when I do it. Further, having staff make these sales—that's what they are—multiplies my efforts, makes my day easier, more fun, more enjoyable, and gives an important extra function to a staff member.

We call all patients by their first name and don't object if they do that with us. We want a warm welcome atmosphere to inspire confidence and to let patients know we love 'em a bunch.

We give patients compliments by the carload: "What a pretty blouse that is, Bertha!" "What a handsome belt buckle, George!" "Hey, Billy, you've got new boots!"

We touch our patients on the shoulder, pat them on the arm, even pat their heads. "Gee, you're a good patient, Ellen!" We even say that when they aren't. It is amazing how patients will later try to earn such praise. It is also touching to see the gratitude in their eyes when we pat their egos.

When something hurts, we say, "I'm sorry." Our concern usually produces a response like, "That's okay, Doc." Or we ask, "I'm sorry, Diane. Can you handle it?" "Oh sure." And they do because they know we truly care.

When we do something without charge, even if my assistant knows it is n/c, I make a point to tell my assistant in a voice the patient clearly hears, "Don't charge for that procedure, Shirley."

I once told my staff that our Governor was going to be a new patient the following week. "What shall we do to get ready for him?" I asked.

"Nothing!" was their prompt reply. No other answer would have been acceptable. For if we have to do something different for a VIP, then we are practicing two-level health care. We love *all* our patients, not just the VIP's. Every patient gets a full measure of our loving care.

I am violently opposed to a form of health-care service that is frequently practiced. I call it *abandon health care*. A patient is brought into the treatment or exam area and then left alone for a long period of time.

Nothing good can happen with a patient stuck alone in an inner room. From the moment they leave their coffee, tea, or hot chocolate cup in the reception room until they are delivered to the appointment and collection crew, no patient is ever alone in our office. They *know* we care.

When patients sit alone, they conjure up all sorts of anxieties about fear, cost, and pain. Further, they usually resent being "dumped." Like I say, nothing good happens when a patient sits alone in a dentist's seemingly threatening environment. So a pleasant, gregarious staff member—they are chosen with those two qualities uppermost—sits and visits with the patients.

Their visiting consists mostly of questions and thoughtful listening. They learn things to tell me when I arrive at the chair. They have an opportunity to allay fear. They discuss fees, when appropriate, to let the patient plan how he will discharge his responsibility to us. They explain procedures. They sell. In short, everything good can happen when my staff babysits our patients.

Patients come in all shapes, colors, and sizes. Ours come from every strata of society because we never have refused to treat a patient who sought our care. Nor have we refused to see a patient who claimed an emergency need on the day he called—never ever.

For us, these are inviolate rules. They're just like our rule that says we will never deny anyone care because of lack of money. We do it because we love people and feel an obligation to care for all who seek our services. And that includes the welfare patients who make up roughly 7% of our practice.

A telephone survey that we conducted revealed that half my colleagues refuse to treat welfare patients. I know all the reasons that are given: welfare patients cheat, they break appointments, they don't take care of the dentistry, and welfare pay schedules are lousy.

While I was in graduate college, I was once on welfare for a short time. Perhaps I have an appreciation for hardship that some of my colleagues do not. Still, I think it is unfair to write off 21 million Americans simply because they haven't had the opportunity or the good fortune we dentists are privileged to enjoy. We will continue to love our welfare patients, just as we do our private patients.

If a patient becomes dissatisfied with our service, a sign in the reception room says it all, "We Guarantee Your Satisfaction!" That's right—we *guarantee* the patient's satisfaction! This, of course, is professional heresy. We were taught in school to only guarantee an effort not a result. To which I say, "We were taught wrong."

What will you not do to satisfy a patient? Remake, repair, replace, and anything you can to make it work? Of course, you will. Think about it for a minute. Your salvage efforts are a guarantee of your result. So why not capitalize on that fact and announce it on the front end?

If a patient simply cannot be pleased by us, we promptly refund any payment made—in full. We do that to defuse him. Here, again, is my guarantee to you: Please a patient and they *may* tell someone; displease a patient and they *will* tell someone. Guaranteed.

The patient I cannot please, I have obviously displeased. If I take one dollar from him, it could be the worst dollar ever taken for it was not earned. But, if I return his dollar, I've taken away his thunder—in effect, I've defused his wrath and weakened his story so much that the odds are strong he won't bad-mouth me.

These are some of the rules of our practice. These rules program our patients to accept our advice. Not every person buys all we have to offer, nor does everyone buy all our rules. We know we cannot possibly please everyone.

But those who do accept us are programmed to respond in concert with our program. When that happens, everyone comes up a winner.

I Love My Profession

When all these good things are going for us, when love abounds at home, with staff, and with our patients—I mean, a caring, thoughtful, committed kind of love—then there is no way we cannot love the beauty of our profession. We cannot help but be happy doing what we are trained so well to do.

And we will love our patients all the more.

A program that includes PASSION! can create a fulfillment of life, which is a stranger to most human beings. That we are fortunate enough to have the opportunity to serve, to express our concerns for other people through our skills and training is truly a blessing.

Live life fully, with PASSION!

20 PROGRAM TO KEEP SCORE

There is little you can learn from doing nothing.

Somehow we have to keep track of our progress with our program. Certain measures are important to use in checking the health of our practice. Certain measures seem needless. We try to choose those measures that give us a quick overview of how well we're doing, without bogging us down with too much accounting gobbledygook. In materials I've read about measuring a practice, there appears to be unnecessary labor induced into what I feel should be natural birth.

I don't care to know how much production I have had per chair hour of practice. I don't care to know how much production I've lost due to cancellations and broken appointments. I am *not* a machine and will *never* work at 100%! I also don't care to know how many crowns or impactions I've served during the month. Perhaps I should care; I just don't.

Maybe someone will convince me one day that those are important numbers to know. My mind is open. Show me. Until then we'll struggle along with more mundane numbers that really tell us something useful—things we must keep abreast of to detect trends. Trends are more useful to our thinking than short-term results.

Other frequently viewed numbers that I *do not* wish to know are: The number of patient visits per month; the average length of patient visits; the average dollar amount of a statement sent; the cost of obtaining a new patient; the exact production per new patient; and the percentage breakdowns of where our business stems from (welfare, insurance, private, and the like). That's enough. There no doubt is more that I don't feel that I need answers for, but lets visit about what we do, not what we don't do. First, one more point.

Before we discuss measures we feel are important to review regularly, there's another old saw that's as useful as most cliches: "Nobody ever got rich in dentistry."

Sadly, I believed that for too many years, which probably was why I lost into six digits on various outside schemes. Those losses inspired me to reassess dentistry, to create a new philosophy, and to challenge other old supposed truisms that I mentioned earlier.

Today, I refuse to let those past losses reprogram my present goals and attitudes. It would be simple to brood, cuss, and mope about them. I can't even tell you the schemers' names, who I allowed to con me into such illusory (and totally elusive) visions of largesse that never would be. They are fully programmed out of my present thoughts, and except for this writing I never discuss them; it would be pointless.

There are thousands of dentists who have gotten rich—past ordinary wealthy—in dentistry. This does not include those who have parlayed practice wealth into other outside investment wealth.

If this book could leave you with only one pearl worth the price, it would be to redirect your attention back to scoring in dentistry rather than looking afield with longing. You would have missed the greatest opportunity of all time and written a sad epitaph for your professional pursuits. But back to our measures.

My main concern with my programming is to improve my net worth. In other words, at the end of the year I expect my net worth to have increased over last year's net worth. If that happens I'm happy. That was why I learned and risked and devoted a year of my life to a program of PASSION! That's my concern as a business person.

Of course, I hope to contribute to people's health, welfare, and happiness along the way. The Great Scorer is keeping track of those measures for me, so except for being sure I do them, I can neither measure them effectively nor interpret the results. How'm I doing, God?

To check my progress, I simply update my net-worth statement. Bill, my banker, appreciates seeing those updates to reinforce his very astute and wise decision to loan me lots of other people's money, of which he is trustee (the bank's bucks). I had to put this paragraph in because I will probably want to borrow more of "his" money next month.

I update it every six months and for sure every year. The update is checked against past statements. I look for growth in hard assets, growth in liquidity, and growth in self-liquidating debt. Those measures tell me how financially stable I am, how much adverse weather I could ride out, and how much progress I've made in the past year.

Net worth is the real bottom line; net profit really isn't. Liken net profit to cattle feed and growth of net worth to how many pounds the cattle put on that year, and you will see the relation of these two numbers. Having fat cattle is more marketable than having a silo full of feed.

On the first of each month my staff members lay various reports on my desk. They tell me figures for the prior month and year to date (YTD). They are:

Production
Production per producer (3 doctors, 3 hygienists)
Collections
New patients
Aging of accounts receivables
Lab production
Hygiene production
Patients who have left the practice
Calls on the InfoLine (see Chapter 11 on Marketing)

In a few minutes I have these digested and scored on a simple score sheet. Here's what I look for in these numbers:

1. *Production.* Did we produce more (or less) than this month last year? Is our YTD production over last year to this point? How much? I expect a minimum of 7% growth.
2. *Production per producer.* How are other profit producers doing in relation to what they have done in the past? I expect them to grow if they are interested in being on our team.
3. *Collections.* Monthly collections can be misleading. YTD collections are far more meaningful. We are hanging in there on the magic 96%.
4. *New patients.* Are we holding our goal of a new patient for every hour the practice is open? Are they coming more from satisfied patients than from marketing devices? I expect a 60:40 ratio. I cannot tell you why I expect that percentage, except to note that satisfied patient referrals tell us we are delivering quality dental experiences. In my view, that is a healthier way to generate new patients in terms of insurance for the future of our practice.
5. *Aging of accounts receivables.* I check the total, wanting it to be no more than my expectation, which is 1.2 times the previous month's production. I also check the 90-day and over receivables to see if my staff is calling them all and following up with our series of three collection letters. When receivables reach that stage, we write off the smaller stuff (below $25) and note that on patients' charts.
6. *Lab production.* I multiply this by commercial lab costs, multiply that number by 30%, and expect the result to not exceed lab employees' salaries.
7. *Hygiene production by hygienist.* This report includes the hygienist's salary. It also includes her salary divided into her production, which does *not* include X-rays. I expect this number to be 3.5 or better. A hygienist who does not produce three times her salary is losing money. One who is producing over 3.5 times her salary three months in a row is due a raise.
8. *Patients who have left the practice.* A finding of our recall assistant. I look through every chart and refer it to the producer who last had a significant office encounter with

this patient. If we are to learn from our mistakes, we have to see those mistakes. Although staff doctors often help each other out on patient problems ("I have an ache now, can someone else see me?"), it is always best to see one's own postop sequelae. It is much too valuable a learning experience to lose.

9. *Calls on the InfoLine.* I like to know how many patients my answering service referred to us from this source and how many calls we had on each of the nine tapes. These data have no special significance, except to help me in the future if I want to change the tapes. It is also of some help in showing me what areas of interest appeal to people. By knowing this I can fashion more useful 5-second phrases for our Time and Temperature community service.

There's another report I look for every Friday: our employee suggestion box. I then report the suggestions in a staff notice and answer them. At the end of each month I award $5 to the best suggestion and $2 to runners-up. My employees have generated some excellent suggestions.

Once in awhile I spot check time cards to see if time is being counted fairly and to see if employees are arriving in sufficient time to be ready for work.

I would have a time clock if I had but two employees. The reason is basic. Two employees will not arrive and depart at the same instant. If they are both paid a daily, weekly, or monthly salary, a dissenting chord is struck by the one who arrives later than the other. "How come Betty earns just as much as I do and gets to waltz in late?" is the silent question always posed.

Or, if you asked an employee to do something extra ("Marcia, would you stay and change the X-ray solution tonight?"), she very naturally feels put upon. A time clock and hourly pay resolve these differences: "Your pay begins when you arrive and extends until you leave." Simple and hassle-free.

Time cards help us assure that we do not exceed the federal eight-hour day and 40-hour week maximums before time and a half begins. The time card is my proof.

A former employee once claimed unemployment compensation after I discharged her. With time cards in hand I was able to prove to the examiner that she had been tardy 94 times in the six months of her employment. Her request was denied, which helped my contribution rate to remain lower following that incident.

I won't spend time discussing all the popular measures of a practice that we ignore. Those we use, I feel, give all we need to know to administer our programs in as simple a manner as possible.

Monthly profit and loss statements are your accountant's dream and produce little information of value, in my view. Same with cash-flow charts and futuristic projections of either. Both can be phoneyed far too easily to be useful.

A breakdown of services rendered is a puzzle to me. What have I learned if I know we did 18% surgery, 61% crown and bridge, and 21% operative? Nothing that I can think of.

I wouldn't use that information to set fees: "Doctor, since you did 50 crowns last month, if you raised the fee $20 per crown, you will earn an extra thousand next month." Oh, yeah? Just maybe I'll do *half* as many since I might price myself out of the market.

Neither would I use that information to exhort staff: "Okay, folks, we were down in C&B production last month; let's pump it up this month." Please tell me no one is so callous as to make that plea.

The same for salaries as a percentage of production, for example. To keep that figure in a reasonable 22–25% category, all we have to do is improve production. I may glance at that figure yearly, but to brood over it monthly is not a sensible game.

As I look through the score cards that we produce, I get a pulse of the practice, a feel for trends that may point out problems. For example, are we collecting at least 30% at the front desk? This I get from the collections report. It's a number that I feel is a fair measure of a proper job both in the reception area as well as at chairside.

Chairside DA's must lay numbers on patients so patients have time to think about how they will discharge their financial responsibilities to us. If that isn't being done, it often results in lowered front-desk collections. By the same token, front-desk staff has to ask for a collection for it to occur.

Naturally, the question is posed the same way we pose all questions to our patients: "Will this be cash, check, or do you prefer to use a credit card?" We offer Mastercard, Visa, and American Express. The question is *not:* "Would you like to pay your balance today?"

That question too easily allows a "no" answer. When "no" is a difficult choice to bring up, as in the first question, it occurs less frequently.

"Would you like your recall appointment in the morning or afternoon?" produces more affirmative answers than "Would you like to make your recall appointment now?" That question is too easily answered "no."

There is one more report that captures my interest, certainly as much as these others. It is the staff report to me on how the practice is faring and their view of it.

In the fall I submit five pages of questions to the staff. These questions focus on all areas of the practice. Some answers are relative value answers, answered with excellent, good, fair, poor. Some answers are yes/no. Some are essay answers. None of the questionnaires is signed by staff.

I learn scads of information from these reports. I collate their answers to see trends; then I report these trends, plus my response to their significance, back to the staff. They appreciate knowing that we care enough to want their opinions.

Last year, a great deal of staff comment concerned fringe benefits. Part of that was my failure to communicate the extent and value of existing fringe benefits. Part of that stemmed from some weaknesses we had in our fringe benefit program.

From that came a five-page fringe benefit booklet to distribute to staff and to use as a tool when we interview prospective employees. We have established a pension and profit-sharing plan as a result of those comments. Staff now know that their views have value, will be heard, and importantly, acted upon for their interest as well as for the good of the office.

An earlier staff questionnaire revealed a problem in presenting our office policies to new patients. It was during a time when we first were enjoying accelerated growth. An office brochure and policy statement arose from that comment. Now, when a new patient arrives, he can be invited into our practice as painlessly as we can devise it, with minimal employment of staff time.

A common theme throughout this book has been a heavy reliance on staff: to make sales, to teach new staff members, to keep me apprised of changes or potential problems in the office, to keep happy while working in a pleasant environment, to communicate with again and again in every way possible. How do we find these gems beyond price? We advertise in the want ads and accept referrals from existing staff. Our want ads simply list our telephone number and some snappy language to excite interest in calling us. It also contains qualifiers, such as "experienced," "night staff hours," "chairside," or whatever we seek.

Their first call is their first interview. How do they come across to the answering receptionist? If they can put together two or three reasonable sentences and qualify for the job, they are invited in to fill out an application and have a two-minute interview. The receptionist notes their name and rates their call in her words: "sounds pleasant," "seems eager," "not too friendly," and the like.

When they show up for an interview, the receptionist again rates them in the same fashion. They fill out our applicant form, I'm informed, and between patients or during a lull I call them back for an interview. We are all looking for an attractive person with a good personality who fulfills our qualifiers. We can judge that personality in seconds because that is exactly the way patients judge our office when they judge an employee.

When several potential employees are ready for final interview, that will take 10 minutes or so. I'm looking for weaknesses that might show up later as problems. They read our employee benefits book, get a tour of the office, and are asked to call back the next day with questions they might have forgotten. Then we hire and put new employees on a three-week trial.

I always call all references. Odd how some applicants list names of people as references who have nothing good to say about the person.

During the trial period they have the right to quit at any time of any day. By the same token I have the right to dismiss at any time of any day. They sign a release that says that and have their husband, father, mother, or someone else close to them sign it, too. It prevents possible future misunderstanding.

We don't always hit. In the past few years, despite weeding efforts, we've had to weed 40 or 50 more who had begun with us. But those who remain are the creme de la creme, the best of the best. They know it is a privilege to work for Dental East. I know it is my privilege to work with them.

One more time: All the reports I receive consume no more than a few minutes of administration time. Staff is alert to what I am looking for. Often, they volunteer the problem before I detect it in our trend reports. Better yet, they often help me with a solution or several suggestions before I have had a chance to address the problem.

Finally, monitoring our programs is a special program of its own. A program where we know the rules we want followed, we execute them, and we do so with PASSION!

You can, too.

21
PROGRAM FOR SELF-PROTECTION

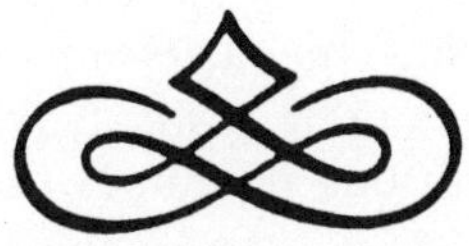

Jenning's Corollary: *The chance of bread falling with the buttered side down is directly proportional to the cost of the carpet.*

Some call it the price of success. But having studied this book to this point, you and I know it for what it really is—it is simply an attempt by others to have their program override ours. Sometimes we let them.

> Doc, you've heard of the Juvenile Alcoholics Achievers program in our town, haven't you? Of course. Well I represent the selection committee, and we've searched the city for a sensitive, intelligent, prominent, respected, and esteemed citizen, someone everyone looks up to, someone everyone loves, someone everyone recognizes to be the epitome of success, solidarity, and caring professionalism, and do you know what, Doc? Each one of us on the committee came up with your name, without the others even knowing about it! Isn't that an incredible coincidence?

Unless your ego needs these trips, you will have to be inventive to talk your way around them. They will happen. And the more successful you become, the more frequent—and urgent—will be the pleas.

Does chairing the fundraiser for the Juvenile Alcoholics Achievers really help your practice? Not a whit. Let no one tell you otherwise.

First, you will alienate all who don't believe in JAA—and there are many in your community who don't. Second, half of the community will see your role for what it really is: self-aggrandizement. Third, the committee members are already patients of other dentists in town. And fourth, publicity for JAA is met by the community at large with one enormous yawn. Who cares about JAA?

Substitute anything you wish for JAA. They're all the same. Do them if you wish, but don't think you will get a boost to your practice by letting JAA reprogram twenty-nine of your evenings with inane meetings.

If you decide to accept such offers, the trick is to give of yourself in such a manner that won't deter your own program.

> Okay, Dan, I'll chair your JAA drive. But I've a few personal rules. First, my schedule has no room for meetings. Second, I want to read and approve anything that goes out with my name on it—before it goes out. Third, I will not make any phone calls or badger any of my friends or colleagues to contribute to JAA. Now, if you still want to use me on those terms, that would be acceptable. If you want more, I guess I'm not your man.

If an inviter can make rules for you—"Doc we want to do this and this and that"—then you have a perfect right to let him know your rules. You may not get the juicy civic plum, but you also will lose no respect, sleep, or time over a program that likely will eat into yours. Remember these:

No committee ever did anything significant.
Every job takes five times longer than it seems.
No truly successful practice was ever built by a community

A lot of this flies in the teeth of the old saw that says you must pay your community rent. Of course, but do it on your terms.

How did I learn these priceless truths? By doing every one of them.

I did them all. My curriculum vitae for civic activities is longer than a giraffe's tail. But those activities didn't build my practice, my family relationships, or my self-esteem. Each of them short-circuited the one thing I know how to do best—practice dentistry.

And when I got down to business and stayed on my program without straying into other pastures, exciting and wonderful things began to happen. It can for you, too.

Two more reprogrammers are at work that we should talk about as we wind down this work so you can wind up yours: the problem patient and the IRS.

Recently I heard a patient swearing at an assistant in an adjacent operatory. There'd been a similar episode with this man before. I went to the operatory and said:

"Leonard, your language is unacceptable to us. We will no longer work for you. Please leave at once."

I raised the chair arm and guided him past the rest of the patients and staff to his coat in the reception room. As he went, he loudly swore with about every four-letter word that has ever steamed a steamy locker room.

We've invited others out of our practice, too. It simply clears the air and gets us back on our program. People with foul mouths deserve foul dentistry, and we simply don't know how to deliver it. We refuse to try.

People who unjustly harangue my staff get the same one-way invitation. People who lie to me ("I did not approve of this denture on tryin!") are also invited out. People who refuse to honor their financial commitments are never allowed back until their old balance is first cleared.

I dismissed an elderly gentlemen the other day who I simply could not please with a new denture. He claimed that it didn't fit tightly enough. He admitted he could eat whole apples with it, but that wasn't good enough! After a dozen denture "adjustments" I simply gave up and refunded his payment in full. I slept very well that night.

The customer is **not** always right!

There's one more problem we all share—the IRS. The IRS would like to reprogram the residue of my yearly efforts into its bottomless coffers. I employ some very astute folks to make sure as little of that occurs as is legally possible.

Any practice that is not incorporated, that does not have a pension and profit-sharing plan in force, that does not have IRA's operable, and that does not maximize legitimate tax shelters is one that is listening to some very bad advice. This book does not have the space to get into these areas, but you have a duty to yourself, your family, and your heirs to hire experts to fashion a course that will salvage some of the fruits of your labor.

There's really little more to offer except my passionate wish for your success, however you define it, with PASSION!

A man once prayed, "Lord give me what I want, but make me want what I should have."

My daughter Cathy once framed a copy of *Footprints* for me. I have found it valuable in fashioning a philosophy that is consistent with PASSION! Let it be the final thought I will share with you.

Do it with PASSION!

Footprints

One night a man had a dream. He dreamed he was walking along the beach with the Lord. Across the sky flashed scenes from his life. For each scene he noticed two sets of footprints in the sand: one belonging to him and the other to the Lord. When the last scene of this life flashed before him, he looked back at the footprints in the sand. He noticed that many times along the path of his life there was only one set of footprints. He also noticed that it happened at the very lowest and saddest times in his life. This really bothered him and he questioned the Lord about it. "Lord, you said that once I decided to follow you, you'd walk with me all the way. But I have noticed that during the most troublesome times in my life, there is only one set of footprints. I don't understand why, when I needed you most, you would leave me." The Lord replied, "My precious,

precious child, I love you and I would never leave you. During your times of trial and suffering, when you see only one set of footprints, it was then that I carried you."

—Author Unknown

EPILOGUE

Robert J. Ringer's book, *Looking Out for #1,* has been villified as a hedonist's handbook. It isn't. People who call it that have probably read no more than its title. And that certainly *sounds* hedonistic.

In like manner, there will be critics who will cry that *3 Steps to the Million-Dollar Practice* is the doctor's hedonistic handbook. It isn't. But to a casual observer, it may sound hedonistic.

To a layman, a million-dollar practice is fantasy land. To a doctor it is nothing more than an opportunity for a fair return on a life committed to the acquisition of skills and knowledge.

In the first place, a million-dollar practice doesn't mean a million dollars of spendable income. It means enormous overhead, enormous responsibility to staff and patients, and healthy "contributions" to the IRS.

In the second place, enormous risks are incurred: in dollar outlay to stock such an operation, in competition from other doctors, in competition from businessmen who enter the field under the generic "retail" health-care concepts, in competition from self (alcoholism, suicide, and divorce statistics support that), in competition from lawyers who look on the professions as "deep pockets" in which to plunge, in competition from personal disasters that can wipe out a life's pursuit in an instant, and in competition from slick businessmen who prey on doctors with scheming regularity.

There need be no apology for anyone maximizing his potential—especially when he does so through delivering the benefits of abundantly healthful living, with care and concern, and does so by providing affordable health care at both reasonable and unreasonable hours.

Those who have the disciplines to marshall a programmed method to successful living need plaudits, not scorn.

This book came about through the application of the principles of programming. First, Steve overcame my former program: The one that did not include the sweat, strain, struggle, and mental discipline required to give birth to these thoughts in writing. It is fairly simple to tell someone your views. But when you must write them out, simplicity becomes complexity.

Steve programmed me to the effort by his persistence. It became easier to do it and get him off my back, than to not do it and endure the burr that he'd placed under my saddle.

Second, the three steps to achieve occurred exactly as outlined in the book.

1. *Know the rules.* The rules in this instance meant reading, studying, thinking, and learning how to express myself with the written word.
2. *Willingness to risk.* Was I willing to take a chance of falling flat on my tokus? A reluctant yes.
3. *And PASSION!* in completing the task. It would have been more comfortable to make it a life project, dawdling along at a relaxed pace, talking about it a lot, but never trying to really complete the project. I established a time goal, restructured my sleep habits, arose very early, and wrote before going to work.

Whether or not the book "works" remains to be seen. But whether or not the book works is not nearly so important as whether or not the programming system works.

It works.